HEALTH AND DEVELOPMENT

HEALTH
AND
DEVELOPMENT

Edited and Presented by
KEVIN M. CAHILL, M.D.

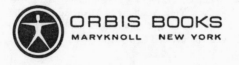
ORBIS BOOKS
MARYKNOLL   NEW YORK

Some of the papers in this volume were first presented in a symposium sponsored by the Tropical Disease Center, Lenox Hill Hospital, New York City, and the Merck Company Foundation, Rahway, New Jersey, and subsequently published in the Bulletin of the New York Academy of Medicine, May 1975.
The essay by Denis Goulet first appeared in *Christianity & Crisis*, May 26, 1975. Copyright 1975 Christianity and Crisis, Inc.

Ad
H.O.C.

CONTENTS

Introduction

KEVIN M. CAHILL, M.D., D.T.M. & H. (LOND.)

Director, The Tropical Disease Center
Lenox Hill Hospital
New York, N.Y.

Professor of Tropical Medicine
The Royal College of Surgeons in Ireland
Dublin, Ireland

HEALTH AND DEVELOPMENT represents a distillate and a departure. Reflected in the theme and choice of topics in this symposium are the experiences derived from Calcutta epidemics, from an Egyptian fever hospital where a simple but fatal syndrome—infant diarrhea—accounts for half the pediatric deaths, from the remote African bush where the game of survival is played out with the rarest participation of trained medical personnel, and from the crises of a Nicaraguan earthquake where the survivors of the disaster may well have envied the dead.

Few who have not experienced the burden of disease and poverty in the Third World can even comprehend its scope or understand its impact on every form of human endeavor. How should one express in living words the anguish implied in a cold statistic such as an infant death rate of 350 to 400 per 1,000 live births in almost any developing land versus an average 12 per 1,000 in the United States? How does one capture for those who have not seen and do not know them the constant pangs of hunger, the dwindling strength of a parasitized parent who wants to work, the pain of unnecessary illness, the frustrations of ignorance, and the unacceptable but almost inevitable loss of every human dream and desire at an early age when individual pleasure and productivity as well as national development should be at the maximum?

The physician has a privileged position from which to view this scene, but alone he is almost impotent to effect any change. For too long medical professionals have spoken only to one another—documenting the toll of disease, studying its causes and victims, calling upon

anyone and everyone to listen to their advice. They have failed, however, to move beyond the traditional limitations of the profession, failed
to realize that merely convincing—or is it conversing with?—one another
has not altered economic policies or significantly influenced political
will, and it is in these arenas that the critical decisions which determine
the extent, or even existence, of health programs are made most frequently. Too rarely have competent, respected health experts been
willing to venture from their safe havens into the turbulent councils
where government priorities are established and financial allocations
are set. Those best qualified have made too small a contribution to these
councils in regard to the human resource, the human potential for, and
the impact on people from developmental projects. Yet all give lip
service to these as the goals of modernization and "progress."

There is a paucity of professional courage in this area, a reluctance
to abandon the rigid, privileged positions of the consultant for the new
but obviously necessary challenges of political decision-making; there
is a poverty of medical initiative, innovation, and even thought. If there
has been a sense of outrage at the human condition in many parts of
the world those who should be most able to express this have been
either unable or unwilling in comprehensible terms which can alter the
opinions and actions of the decision-makers noted above to articulate the
harsh realities of life as they exist for the majority of mankind.

For too long we who deal with and know most intimately the one
unique resource of the Third World—the human being—have allowed
our projects to remain dreams and our priorities to be words. No
international health worker is blind to the obvious interdependence of
health, education, agriculture, engineering, and so many other disciplines, but need we wait for simultaneous progress in all these fields
before any change is made? That approach seems, at best, an exercise in
futility and perverse sophistry and, at worst, an admission of predictable
failure, an excuse for no new action, and a defense of the deplorable
present status of international health.

Any perceptive worker in this field realizes that the challenges of
tropical medicine today are not merely a repetition of the great era
of defining new parasites and life cycles, of discovering effective modes
of individual therapy, or even of mass methods for the control of
infectious diseases. Instead, he must deal with the reality that health
services reach less than 10% of the population in most developing

countries, that the world population is expanding faster than its health services, that malnutrition is the rule for two thirds of all mankind, and that in the developed nations there seems to be neither the political will, the money, nor the technology to alter this course.

There has been, in fact, a growing—if long overdue—appreciation that transferring Western medical technology, systems, and approaches to developing lands may not only be a great waste of funds, talent, and equipment, but is often an absolute detriment to an effective and appropriate health-delivery service. In Somalia, for example, I have noted the lasting burden of an inappropriate health "gift" when that poor East African nation attained her independence.[1] The European Economic Community (EEC) presented to that nation of nomads an ultramodern hospital—a building that belonged in Brussels. The structure almost reduced the nation's health budget to the breaking point while also centralizing almost all medical services in the capital city. The hospital may have served the wealthy few, but the nomadic masses suffered more neglect. The challenge of redefining the education and role of the physician and the auxiliary health worker has been considered in an earlier program in this series.[2]

New challenges exist not only in health but in all areas of development. At one time it was de rigueur to define individual and national development in income per capita and in levels of gross national product (GNP). In the field of tropical medicine one could even calculate a "malaria tax," which referred to the extra cost of a product due to inefficiency and illness caused by that disease. Gradually, however, these terms became mere words to the newly independent nations struggling to define their own identities. Once again lip service was not enough.

Many of these new nations had virtually one resource only—their citizenry. Political and economic leaders had to grapple with the less specific but more real human factors of life itself, health, satisfaction, pride, personal and national achievement, and a myriad of other investments and dividends that defied standard classifications. Nations began to recognize that modernization was not necessarily synonymous with development and that the most desired so-called improvements were often accompanied by unexpected, disastrous complications.

I have cited this *Symposium on Health and Development* as a personal and professional distillate and departure. My own work has evolved from the study of distinct tropical infections and the use of mass-screening techniques to a wider consideration of medicine as a vehicle for international cooperation and understanding. The present work extends that thesis while making more specific the necessity for involving the politician, diplomat, and financier if improvement in health care is to be our true goal.

We must no longer merely give lip service to independence and nationalism, but must consider their adverse effects as proper matters for our consideration if we really hope to make effective changes. Can we continue, in the handwashing fashion of Pontius Pilate, to give lip service to the ideals of the World Health Organization (WHO) without facing the hard fact that its total annual expenditure is less than one tenth of New York City's health budget, that the WHO is only an advisory body that does not claim operational activities in most health areas in the tropics, and that the WHO is an organization whose member states have been known to deny the very presence of cholera for fear of losing tourist income. This should not be misinterpreted as unfair criticism of the WHO—the organization does serve a number of unique functions—but to cite the danger of continuing to indulge in vacuous compliments as an alternative to facing facts and dealing realistically with them.

We must deal with the ethical problems of development and recognize political and economic priorities if an improvement in health is to be our real goal. If we remain within the confines of academia or take refuge from reality behind the privileges of our profession we cannot hope—and do not deserve—to have a significant impact on the future health of our species.

This is the 10th in a series of symposia[2-4] inaugurated shortly after I returned from residence in the tropics. There have been six detailed dissertations on specific disease entities, an historical review, an examination of health education for the tropics, and a philosophic program, *The Untapped Resource*,[3] which considers the relations between medicine and diplomacy. That volume was translated into a proposed statute in the United States Congress, the International Health Agency Act of 1971, and provided the basis for extensive hearings in both the Senate and House of Representatives on the role of the United States in world health. The hearings did not reveal a flattering picture, and the bill did not pass into law, but at least senators and representatives were informed, most for the first time; there had been no Congressional hearings on international health in more than 15 years and the declining medical programs of the Agency of International Development (AID) were virtually unknown by those who annually allocated the funds.

The possibility of moving a philosophy of medicine into Congressional hearings and of drawing upon the goodwill that is available to our profession (if we are willing to venture forth with sound ideas) further stimulated the present program.

There is great benefit in having the secretary-general of the United Nations (UN) open a symposium on health and development in the world. But Kurt Waldheim's contribution is more than the expected token benediction; it forcefully cites the ideals of the UN and the WHO while clearly noting lapses in political will and the fragility of international cooperative efforts.

The necessity for political understanding and will to implement any significant health program in a developing country is discussed by Sr. Eduardo Frei, the former president of Chile. Widely respected as among the most thoughtful and articulate government leaders in Latin America in this century, Sr. Frei cites the priority that health care may assume among the competing goals of a developing nation, but notes the realities that often determine the final balance of an inadequate economy.

In a poetic paper Lord Ritchie-Calder discusses the ethical and economic implications of health-development projects. Few men have had so vast an experience in interpreting for the public the advances of science and technology as this Scottish Lord whose career has taken him from the political front lines of the Labour Party through journalistic endeavors on five continents to several academic appointments as a professor of international relations and presently to the philosophic post of senior fellow at the Center for Democratic Studies in California.

For almost 20 years Professor W. H. Russell Lumsden was director of the Sleeping Sickness Services in East Africa. While making major contributions to the science of tropical medicine, he has had an almost unique vantage point from which to observe the effects of nationhood on the diseases of a region where insect vectors do not recognize political borders. He was the director of research programs under the relatively uncomplicated Colonial Medical Service during the period of transition and under the new African leadership. He has had extensive experience with the problems of maintaining a health and research service during periods when expatriated personnel did not have the security of a home-employment base and before adequate numbers of indigenous medical leaders existed. His paper is solid, reflective, and realistic, yet optimistic.

The public record of the Hon. Hugh L. Carey is ennobled by a long-standing and effective commitment to the improvement of health care. Throughout his long career in the House of Representatives Mr. Carey provided critical political leadership in this country for global medicine and, almost alone, focused attention on this country's declining role in what he called "the one war we can win," the worldwide battle against disease. He introduced the International Health Agency Act of 1971 in Congress. His knowledgeable and persuasive paper demonstrates the understanding, encouragement, and conviction of a perceptive political person. He embodies the finest of that critical political facet too long ignored—indeed almost absent—from previous international health conferences.

The interrelations of host, infecting agent, and environment are considered in the presentation of Professor Herbert M. Gilles. His own epidemiologic studies in Africa demonstrate clearly that one cannot be comforted by the facade of modern medical centers, for far too frequently the expected beneficial effects on health statistics prove illusory if not franky deceptive. Certainly they often do not extend far from the building itself. The emergence of new patterns of disease and unrecognized health challenges from so-called developmental programs have formed the substance of many of Professor Gilles' well-known studies in Africa. He emphasizes the complexity of medicine in the developing world and the importance of considering social and economic factors in interpreting the significance and spread of disease, rather than merely establishing the incidence of infection, defining etiologic agents, or measuring the resistance of a host.

Research in tropical medicine has been justified for many years in highly industrialized and developed nations on the premises that these diseases pose a military threat to our armed forces, that they may afflict the small percentage of our citizens who travel through the tropics, or that they may become epidemic once again within our own borders. Alternatively, such research is defended on the basis that the more fortunate few of the world have a moral obligation to assist the disadvantaged many. Without denying the validity of any of these premises, it has long been my belief that research in tropical medicine can be readily justified—and should be financially supported—because the knowledge accrued from studying exotic infections so frequently has a direct bearing on our understanding of common ailments.

One can, for example, think in terms of that most exotic infection, kuru, which is transmitted by cannibalism in the mountains of New Guinea. It is unlikely that such open cannibalism will flourish in the United States, and one might well question the allocations of diminishing research funds to the study of such a syndrome. However, the clear relation of kuru to multiple sclerosis has changed that thinking, and the investigation of many latent, slow viral infections has been elucidated by studies begun in the mountains of New Guinea. The entire field of cancer research has been greatly stimulated by the detection of an exotic African lymphoma; the epidemiologic and therapeutic implications of these studies are profound. Dr. Joseph H. Burchenal, a world authority on the chemotherapy of cancer, reviews his own and other studies on Burkitt's lymphoma, first described in East Africa, and now recognized as but one of the curable forms in a broad mosaic of disease called cancer that is international in distribution and multifaceted in presentation and—partially because of observations made in rural Africa—no longer sounds the same uniformly ominous note for its victims.

In the past decade almost all emerging nations have carefully scrutinized the role of international cartels in their economies; despite many failures to wed the developed and developing lands, there have been far more successful instances where private investments from capitalistic societies have been able to flourish, even under highly socialistic or rigidly totalitarian regimes. Few men have as successfully developed this bridge of mutual benefit as Mr. G. A. Costanzo, vice chairman of First National City Bank. With a background that includes determining fiscal policies for our State Department, senior positions in the World Bank, and a professorship in economics, Mr. Costanzo now directs the largest American banking firm overseas.

He deals daily with the reality of global monetary interdependence and the necessity of wedding the profit motive of private investment with the goals of a new nation's growth. He has considered the impact of health on economic productivity, and bluntly notes that the major funds for health services in developing countries must emanate from within those lands. Whether one agrees with this philosophy or not, we in the medical field must learn to deal with such facts, plan realistically within such limits, and increasingly involve such financiers in every aspect and stage of international health programs if our projects are to have lasting effect.

We conclude this volume with a contribution by Denis Goulet. Internationally known for his rare blend of idealism and realism, Professor Goulet, in a provocative essay, sees world hunger and world health as challenges to both our political will and our conscience.

Medicine is a noble profession with a long and rich heritage of individual service. At the international level, however, it can no longer function effectively as an isolated discipline and it certainly cannot be viewed as an exercise in charity. It is one of the few common grounds on which those interested in world peace must base their efforts and focus their energies. As was contended in *The Untapped Resource*, medicine, almost uniquely, is the cement of the global community and must be strengthened by politicians, diplomats, economists, and philosophers as well as physicians, if there ever is to be both health and development in this world.

REFERENCES

1. Cahill, K. M.: *Health on the Horn of Africa*. London, Spottiswoode, 1969.
2. Cahill, K. M., editor: *Teaching Tropical Medicine*. Baltimore, University Park Press, 1973.
3. Cahill, K. M., editor: *The Untapped Resource*. Maryknoll, N.Y., Orbis, 1971.
4. Cahill, K. M., editor: *Clinical Tropical Medicine*. Baltimore, University Park, 1972, vols. 1 and 2.

HEALTH IN A WORLD PERSPECTIVE

KURT WALDHEIM

Secretary General
The United Nations
New York, N.Y.

M ANY years ago an American doctor in an Asian country, appalled by the incidence of infant mortality, remarked that this was a terrible tragedy. A member of his staff retorted. "Think how much greater a tragedy it would be if they *didn't* die." The remark was not as heartless or as brutal as it sounds. The staff member knew what the prospects of life were for the surviving children: a desperate struggle against overwhelming odds, no education worth the name, virtually no prospects of employment, and, after all this, a life expectancy of less than 40 years for the most fortunate. The staff member, no doubt unwittingly, put his finger on the key sentence in the Constitution of the World Health Organization (WHO) since it was established in 1948: "Health is a state of complete physical, mental, and social well-being, and not merely the absence of disease and infirmity." In short, the reduction of infant mortality, although obviously highly desirable, is not the solution in itself. The doctor may save a child, but what is he saving him for?

There is now a much greater appreciation of the fact that all the great global problems which we face are interconnected. I can think of no more dramatic single example than that of schistosomiasis, which now affects more than 200 million people. In his speech to the General Assembly of the United Nations on September 23, 1974, U.S. Secretary of State Henry Kissinger pledged "specific proposals" from the United States to control this disease. While this is very welcome, it is important to emphasize that projects to expand water resources in developing countries must be designed to ensure that in distributing water we do not spread this terrible disease further. We have learned a bitter lesson.

We are now groping toward the realization that many of the most intractable health problems are closely linked to factors of the environment, life-styles, urban tensions, social customs, and other crucial but hitherto neglected elements. If one takes a global approach, one is increasingly struck by the vast disparities in the incidences of certain diseases and also by the linkages. To take one example: In El Paso, Texas, the average annual incidence of cancer of the throat among adults is 1.8 per 100,000; in the Gonbad district of Iran it is 206.4 per 100,000 among males, and in females it is even higher. In Normandy and Brittany it is 40 per 100,000, and it is higher in the black communities in the United States. What are the reasons for these disparities and linkages? I speak as a layman, but I suggest that the global experience increasingly emphasizes the profound complexities of health problems and the need to view them in a much wider and deeper social context than in the past.

Since its creation, the WHO has concentrated its efforts—within a relatively small budget—upon the need to control or eradicate communicable diseases. Its most signal triumph has been in smallpox, which in 1967 afflicted 30 nations and now is endemic in only four. In 1967 Sierra Leone, for example, had the world's highest incidence of smallpox; the disease has been eliminated totally there. There are good indications that by the end of 1975 this former scourge may be destroyed. In addition to the human suffering and fear that thus have been eliminated, in the United States this also will mean an annual saving in vaccine and distribution of some $150 million a year—a truly remarkable return on investment, as the annual contribution to the program by the United States over the past 10 years has never exceeded $3 million. Only as a result of this global program has it been possible for the surgeon-general of the United States to advise the states that the routine vaccination of children against smallpox is no longer necessary.

In other fields—notably malaria, cholera, and tuberculosis—the results have also been remarkable but not so spectacular. There is no technical reason why they should not have been equally successful, but administrative, financial, and political factors have become involved. For instance, certain countries which are dependent upon tourism and foreign investment have been reluctant to admit the existence of diseases which would obviously affect these industries; the shortsightedness, not to mention the irresponsibility, of such actions hardly requires comment. The same record as in smallpox could be achieved in these other communicable diseases if the political will were present; the first element of political will is to face facts.

But the most significant and important element in our new approach is to regard communicable diseases as only part of the over-all social and economic problem: i.e., to regard them as products of a deeper problem.

In a recent statement the director-general of the WHO, Dr. Half-dan Mahler, stated with characteristic candor that "the most signal failure of the World Health Organization, as well as of Member States, has undoubtedly been their inability to provide the development of basic health services." This is a criticism which we must take seriously.

By "basic health services" we mean the fundamentals of health care: preventive health care not only for urban populations, which have always been comparatively advantaged, but also for rural populations; clean water; the provision of basic medicines; hygiene; decent standards of living; the disposal of sewage; balanced diets; and knowledge of birth control. We are talking particularly about the availability of such basic health facilities for all. It is our judgment that in the developing countries—where in some areas there is only one doctor to 40,000 people—it is undoubtedly possible to design a health-delivery system that has wide coverage, that the people can afford, and that provides the primary essentials. An example of this is the system developed by the People's Republic of China, which has so impressed observers.

As the recent World Population Conference emphasized, the nation-state must be the executive instrument of health policies, and these must be part of a single strategy. The United Nations has long pioneered in this development, based on the view that this subject must be viewed as a whole. All matters affecting the well-being of the individual must be incorporated into developmental strategies, but health care is self-evidently one of the most crucial areas. We also know that national policies themselves must be part of a global strategy. As we have proved in the case of smallpox, we can achieve this global outlook in the eradication of communicable diseases. It is now imperative that we recognize it in a wider context, in the words of the United Nations Charter, "to promote social progress and better standards of life in larger freedom."

THE POLITICAL REALITIES OF HEALTH
IN A DEVELOPING NATION

EDUARDO FREI

Former President of Chile

I am no specialist in the field of health, but I have had the opportunity to consider the overall problems which a State must meet and therein to duly identify the role which health must play. In other words, I am able to deal with the subject of health and development from a peculiar angle.

The first point that I must stress is that it is quite impossible to make general assertions validly applicable to the various developing nations. This very division of the world into "developed" and "developing" countries is a common simplification which is being rapidly modified. A very wide range may be found within both groups. There is, further, a great distance between the so-called superpowers and the other so-called developed nations.

In turn, substantial differences exist among the developing countries themselves. Some of these enjoy a per capita income of more than one thousand dollars and their rate of illiteracy does not go beyond 6 or 7 percent. Yet, there are others whose income does not reach fifty dollars and whose illiteracy rate exceeds 50 percent.

Nor are these differences merely continental, as would be the case when speaking of Africa, Southeast Asia or Latin America. The degree of evolution varies widely within each of these land masses. If we take the case of Latin America, for example, we can appreciate that within it there are vastly different economic and social levels, as measured by income, education, nutrition, health and other such indices. Hence, the risk in generalized statements or formulas.

Perhaps the only generalization possible is that the health problem should hold a preeminent position in the plans of any State, whether developed or not. If the purpose of development is man himself—as it must be—then his health is one of the utmost priorities, since it is the most essential and direct physical asset of a human being.

The right to health is incorporated in the Universal Declaration of Human Rights of the United Nations and in the Constitutions of many countries. In my own nation, Chile, for instance, the social rights of Health, Welfare, Medical Assistance and Social Service were added to civil rights in 1948.

In the Western hemisphere the Charter of Punta del Este, in 1961, incorporated health as a decisive economic and social factor, and in 1967, at the Meeting of the Heads of State of the Americas, definite commitments were made with this same understanding, going far beyond maternity and child care, which are given special dedication and concern throughout the world.

There is no question, then, of the theoretical basis for the priority of health. The specific point, however, is the actual interpretation of these principles and here—as is usually the case—we meet the real problem.

How may one express, practically, the priority which is given to health? It is obvious that health does not specifically depend only on the direct action of the health services, but also on a number of other factors that contribute to what is known as the standard of living of a community.

It is on the basis of this consideration that one may develop a health policy and assign to it the corresponding priorities that depend not only on direct factors, but, more often than not, on what one might term indirect factors, such as income, housing, nutrition, unemployment, and even geographical and climatic conditions. Can one establish uniform criteria governing these factors without being superficial? I believe this to be rather difficult.

For instance, in the case of a specific community one would have to consider where and how much direct or indirect financial investment is most important and useful. It might well be that investments in education, housing, sanitation, availability of food resources, particularly for children and expectant mothers, would be investments of absolute priority which, although not reflected in the direct health expenditure, do basically affect it. Moreover, direct health investments could, indeed, be useless in the absence of such indirect outlays.

The adjustment of this priority, which requires reflection on the amount of both economic and human investments, is most delicate, inasmuch as it depends on the degree of development of the community. Thus, each State must evaluate how to determine the proportion of direct and indirect investment, although I might dare suggest that in the presence of lower development, indirect investment assumes a higher significance.

As a matter of fact, a publication edited by Dr. Kevin M. Cahill quotes the opinion of Dr. Rene Dubos, which I fully share: Dr. Dubos expresses "a deeply felt conviction that the extent of health improvement that ensues from building ultramodern hospitals with up-to-date equipment is probably trivial in comparison with the results that can be achieved at much lower cost by providing all infants and children with well-balanced food, sanitary conditions, and a stimulating environment."[1]

In addition to these obvious indirect factors that affect health and its priorities, new ones of considerable importance have arisen, such as the pollution of air, water and soil. Therefore, any investment in these fields forms part of that which a State devotes to the welfare of its population.

The improvement of direct health services will be possible only to the extent that the country attains a higher degree of national employment and higher personal income, which in turn may be dependent on environmental, sanitary and nutrition problems as well as the strictly health issues.

Yet, even this apparently obvious statement may have specific modifications. In the particular case of Latin America—as I dare speak only of this continent—the eradication of epidemic and endemic tropical diseases becomes a priority above any other.

This reflection leads us to the question of direct investment, and here again we confront the practical problem of how to determine priorities within the available expenditures. It is essential, therefore, first to analyze the means available to a specific nation with respect to human resources and physical infrastructure.

There are, for instance, countries possessing a good tradition in the formation of medical personnel, but weak with regard to the preparation of ancillary personnel, ranging from nurses, midwives, odontologists to research chemists and even health education experts. A similar situation occurs with infrastructure; it is present in some cases, but is often ineffective because of limited personnel, lack of coordination among institutions devoted to health matters, or the lack of specialized administrators.

The priority put on health is often falsely gauged by the luxury of some hospitals, by the equipment they possess, or by some relatively high-level scientific or professional medical centers; embedded in extraordinarily poor environments, these appear as ancient feudal castles, surrounded by miserable serfs living under precarious conditions.

Such centers are related to and in turn receive incentives from the most highly qualified world centers, engaged in problems that often do not meet the needs of the developing nations or are not concerned with the maladies of the great majority which could be attended to more easily and at a lower cost.

Therefore, these centers cannot meet massive demand and may, indeed, meet only a small demand of very selected individual cases, which seem almost irrelevant in the presence of far greater social needs.

Priorities must evidently be based on efficiency and on the yield of investments, and not on brilliant, though often deceitful, appearances. Certain illnesses that afflict large sectors of the population may be controlled by simple and massive methods, by modest facilities of much greater efficiency operated by personnel whose training does not demand lengthy periods or high costs.

This proposition, however, needs to be properly gauged, for if all health efforts are concentrated on a mediocre massification, mediocrity in all respects might well result.

Therefore, the best formula seems to be a combination of massive public health action with a few highly qualified centers having performance excellence as their target. These latter centers will increase the general level of knowledge and, consequently, of human resources, further allowing them to keep abreast of scientific progress, and through them to impart continued training to the various specialities in their own country. Unfortunately, these centers generally tend to become enclosed, often because of their incapability to set up communication with other sectors located in what we may term labor fronts. This is a basic problem that must be overcome.

In establishing health priorities in any developing country it is essential that this sector not be left to a policy of "laissez faire." It must be a part of the overall planning of all resources and efforts made to carry out the national goals.

If the State and its universities, for example, do not invest in the formation of personnel, are they in a position to demand that their professionals stay for a specific period in rural areas or regions far removed from the urban centers?

May the forming of professionals in each of the various specialized fields, or the issuance of grants within or without the country, be left to chance, or must they be assigned on the basis of clear requirements, tasks and targets?

All this, therefore, leads us to conclude that all the national efforts related to health—including both the public and private sectors—must follow specific planning and not be left either to mere chance or to private initiative alone.

For this same reason, the developing nations must see that every cent invested yields its maximum and that resources are fully utilized.

Such planning should not be conceived as the function primarily of the State or of the technical bureaucracies. In our opinion, the administrative authorities, the medical associations and other professional organizations must also participate, as well as regional representatives of the respective communities, whose cooperation, control and vigilance are essential. The consumers of such services must always be heard; as the word itself denotes, they are the ones who use them and are often the ones that suffer from them. Under these conditions, the allocation of resources within the health sub-sector must establish priorities in line not only with the requirements of the country as a whole, but on regional needs as well.

The first question is always whether it is cheaper to avoid an illness or to cure it—whether the protection and development of health or the recuperation thereof takes first priority. In South America, it must be noted that no matter how sophisticated it may sound to cut funds allocated to the recovery of health in order to divert them to preventative efforts such as the improvement of drinking water, development of sewage disposal, or vaccination campaigns, one must recall that in some developed areas no high incidence, epidemic diseases remain to be controlled through low cost health programs.

In Chile, for example, the greater part of transmissible illnesses have been eradicated: malaria, smallpox, yellow fever, etc. In the Americas, no cases of smallpox have been reported since May 1971 and, in Chile, since 1954. Consequently, it is evident that growing support must be given to health services in the area of rehabilitation and recuperation.

Another equally significant question emerges within this framework. Shall investment be made through the public or the private sector? I am convinced that in countries possessing at least the same degree of development as my own, the massive care of the health of the population is possible only through the public sector. I am fully aware of the danger of bureaucratization, of the tendency to centralization, and of a certain dehumanization in treatment, but I believe that this is nonetheless the most adequate system for best utilizing the resources available to protect and rehabilitate health. This does not exclude a certain degree of free medical practice, or in some population strata a higher mobility to choose the doctor or to combine specific services with a private practice.

It is undoubtedly easier and more feasible to plan for the entire sector in a truly socialized system of medicine, in which the distribution of health is fairer. We must remember, however, that in the developing world the availability of doctors is consistently low. In Latin America, with the sole exception of Argentina, where the relation reaches 22 doctors for every 10,000 people, this ratio fluctuates between 1 and 8 doctors per 10,000 inhabitants (5.8 in the case of Chile). Moreover, it is not only the number of doctors which matters, but also the number of hours which they may devote to the community.

There is the possibility of organizing medical attention in such a way that each doctor could not only serve in the national health system, but also have a private practice. Even better, some systems of social medicine permit the patient to choose his doctor, a situation which could even increase the number of hours devoted to private practice.

For example, if all doctors were to serve in the national system, each one would dedicate no more than 44 hours a week, or possibly less, to State service, and could devote as much time as he chose to his private practice.

If all doctors were to be fully engaged in private practice, higher incomes would obviously be attained. But this means placing medicine in the health market; that is to say, it would be made available only to those who could afford to purchase it. The blunt truth of the matter is that private medicine, or the tendency towards such a solution, leads to the best attention for those sectors enjoying the higher income and to an increasingly deficient one for the lower income sectors.

This represents yet another factor in the imbalance of standards of living and the unfair division of goods and positions so significant in most of the developing nations.

The combination of both socialized and private systems of health care has the advantage, therefore, of ensuring attention to the basic needs of the population, besides substantially increasing the number of medical hours dispensed. This also facilitates financing the services. A practical experiment of this kind was successfully carried out in Chile.

Health planning implies consideration of the most varied problems. I shall refer to only some of them.

Many countries erroneously budget investment in impressive buildings, yet no precise projection is usually made on the cost of maintaining and using such buildings. We need not point out, for instance, that every two years the operational cost of a hospital matches its building cost—to which must also be added the cost of all its equipment.

This is why one sees buildings unused for years either because they lack installations adequate to their size and function, or because they have improperly trained personnel. One also frequently notices the repeated purchase of costly equipment for various medical centers because the initial equipment has been poorly used. In health, as in all other fields, one must coordinate and concentrate scant economic and technical resources.

In my opinion, attention to the availability of medical drugs is of great importance. In nations like my own this expenditure is disproportionate, particularly since drugs and medicines must be purchased abroad from powerful firms that sell their products under their own trademark at very high prices. Thus, both public and private expenditures in the field of health have been very seriously increased by the cost of medications. This is an important consideration—often not sufficiently appreciated, even though it represents major financial outlays for the developing countries.

Allow me to again refer to events in Chile as an example. With the strong support of the Medical School this problem was approached in an effort to rationalize the use of medicines. To this end, a National Formulary was prepared, listing all the essential products by their generic names. The public sector is totally supplied with this line of medicines, produced by a State Laboratory. The private sector—any person—may purchase these same medicines at the drug stores in competition with the respective trademark product.

This measure was taken on the basis that "inasmuch as the supply and administration of medicines is such a determining factor, it is abso-

lutely essential to take all steps leading to complete, timely and continued supply, as well as to allow them to be purchased at a fair price
compatible with the State resources and the needs required to be met."
It is evident that there are many basic, effective and irreplaceable
medicines. However, there are an even greater number of useless
medicines. It has been found that effective therapeutics require a limited number of scientifically chosen drugs. The list of these drugs identified by their generic names and the corresponding pharmaceutical
forms thereof is what was termed the National Formulary.

As a result of this policy, it is now possible to obtain reserpine tablets, for instance, for one-seventh of the cost of the trademark product;
chlordiazepoxide tablets are available at one-third of the trademark
drug; imipramin pills cost one-fifth, and the cloxacilin capsule is available at 50 percent below the trademark price. The foregoing is but one
example of how dramatically the manner of providing drugs and
medicines can affect the cost of providing health care.

Much is said and written today about the transfer of technology as
both a focal point and a condition for development. One of the critical
areas for such a transfer is the field of medicine. The most serious
complications may arise, however, because of the manner in which
medical technology is transferred, because of the dependencies that it
generates, and because of the costs it implies—all of which have a
strong negative impact on the developing countries.

Population growth is another significant element which must be considered, for it affects any kind of health planning as well as any
economic and social analysis of the cost of health programs.

During the decade 1960–1970 the Latin American population growth
rate reached 2.9 percent a year. This is higher than any other rate
registered in the world. In Meso-America—Mexico, Central America
and Panama—it reaches 3.4 percent. In the tropical region of South
America, 3.1 percent; in the Caribbean area, 2.3 percent. In North
America, it is 1.4 percent, and in that part of South America enjoying
a temperate climate, 1.9 percent. The developing countries of this continent show, therefore, the full range of growth rates known in the
world, from the highest to the lowest.

Here again, general assertions are hard to make; I shall restrict myself to our own experience. The family planning program which was
applied in our country was not intended to affect the *size* of the popula-

tion, as its growth rate is 1.9 percent or less. It was directed exclusively to fighting *criminal* abortion; in other words, it was meant to protect the mother, the child and the family group. (The case of those countries whose rates exceed 3 percent is, of course, another matter.) The family planning program was carried out exclusively in the public sector of health and incorporated in the mother-and-child programs.

It is directed to multiparous mothers having serious social and economic problems and particularly to those who have already resorted to abortion. Any final decision in this respect rests with the mother or the couple.

Since in Chile all abortion is illegal, its practice had become generally sought by low economic and social strata expectant mothers to avoid the unwanted child. Maternal death rate is seriously influenced by this cause, and one-third of the maternity beds are taken up by cases of infected abortions due not only to the great numbers but also to the longer period of hospitalization required.

In the ten-year period, this program resulted in bringing down maternal death by one-half, and in decreasing abortion death to one-third.

Within the priorities of any planning, child health has a privileged position. The Charter of Punta del Este, subscribed to by all the countries in the Americas and later ratified by the 1967 Declaration of the Presidents of the Americas, set as a target the reduction of mortality of minors under five years of age to half the present rate.

At the beginning of the sixties, the death rate of children under five years of age in Latin America accounted for 41 percent of the total death roll. Between 1961 and 1969, there was a decrease for those from one to four years of age of 75 percent of the proposed target in Meso-America, and of 81 percent in South America. Barbados, Chile and Peru exceeded the target by having attained an even higher reduction. Similar results were also obtained in decreasing death rates of infants under one year of age. All this reveals how a sound policy can reach evident and quick results.

It is obvious that not all countries have national services entrusted with all health actions for all their populations. Numerous organizations and institutions devoted to this end exist in the countries of this continent; frequently there is a lack of coordination among them, which is a basic cause of the poor performance and an important loss of human and material resources.

Although a single Government Health Service may appear to be the ideal and final solution, it is not an easy matter to create one within a short time. Yet, there is a prior stage that may be approached immediately, and that is a coordination among all organizations concerned with health. This is the process or stage which we have named in Chile the National Health System.

All public sector or social security organizations responsible for health maintain their individual nature, but they must direct their operations under a coordinating council. This helps to avoid duplication of efforts and promises to provide the best service possible to the community. To this end, the National Health Consulting Council was established in 1967, which, among other objectives, set up the Planning and Budget Office, carried out studies on human resources in the health field and on the performance of professionals and the various services, and investigated the economic capacity of the country to absorb the additional demand for services and personnel as well as its future expansion.

The purchase of drugs (National Formulary), of instruments and equipment for all institutions under the Council was also standardized, and a Central Supply Office was established. The Council, with the assistance of outstanding specialists, took up the problem of alcoholism and submitted concrete proposals for an overall government action, including a bill which was presented to the National Congress.

Permanent committees were also set up to deal with cancer, tuberculosis, recuperation and rehabilitation, technical assistance, and fellowships for the specialized training of graduate personnel. These fellowships were granted according to specific requirements for personnel trained in special fields. In addition, highly specialized equipment, such as that used in cancer, was centralized and made available to all institutions.

All this effort, of which we have pointed out only some outstanding aspects, later received significant support from the Pan American Health Organization, which recommended in 1969 "that highest administrative and political level Councils or Health Committees be established with sufficient legal authority to assist the Ministry of Health in the preparation of its policies and in the administrative coordination at an operational level."

In my opinion, the determination of priorities greatly depends on the

philosophy behind the concept of development. If development is really intended to make economic and social growth serve the human
being, then health priority assumes a different meaning. Some believe
that the fundamental question in developing countries is the availability
of labor that will allow, even at the sacrifice of many values, a fast
economic growth that at a second stage will imply a social investment.
I am convinced that such a theory is erroneous. In the world today,
because of factors that would be irrelevant to analyze at this stage, it is
impossible to think of economic development without a parallel social
development—that is to say, a human development. Such development
implies investments in education, in housing, in nutrition, in a special
concern for the child, in sanitary conditions. In one word, I would call
it human investment.

The effort directed to economic development, without which social
development would no doubt be a baseless illusion, must contemplate
the individual as its objective. Individual and collective efforts must
first meet the fundamental demands of the entire community, and they
may not be distorted by the profit that some make for their own benefit, or by the incentive of artificial consumption while others are de-
nied access to even basic nutrition.

Thus understood, overall health assumes a priority which no other
objective may exceed. We must judge the priority given to health not
only by the amounts of money expended, but also by the presence of
techniques which allow—as we have indicated—the best utilization of
all the resources allocated to the health sector. For quite often failure
does not result from a faulty analysis of the problem, but from the
inadequate use of the means available to solve it.

REFERENCES

1. Cahill, K., *The Untapped Resource*
(Maryknoll, New York: Orbis, 1971), pp.
64–65.

A HUMANE MISSION
FOR AMERICAN FOREIGN POLICY

HON. HUGH L. CAREY

Governor, the State of New York

FROM our early days as a nation, dominant American characteristics have included idealism and humanitarian concern. These characteristics have been reflected in our conduct of international health activities. In 1794, the Congress of the United States voted $15,000 for relief of French refugees from Haiti. In 1812, despite the exigencies of war with England, the Congress voted $50,000 for purchase of flour and corn to send to earthquake-devastated Venezuela. Early in the 19th century, there were voluntary efforts in international health such as those of the American doctor, Peter Parker, who went to Canton, China to found an Opthalmic Hospital to serve the poor of that city. From these early modest beginnings, to our major support of UNRRA and later United Nations agencies, of "Point Four" and successor institutions, and of countless voluntary international health programs, we have reaffirmed our dedication to helping to bring health to other nations.

The long years of the Vietnam War, however, have brought an erosion of confidence and purpose. In the aftermath of the oil crisis and inflation of raw material prices, we have come to preoccupy ourselves with the plight of rich countries, rather than poor. Recession and unemployment have left us with too little attention for the impoverished and starving, who constitute the majority of mankind. Where the spirit of community service and international idealism once swept across university campuses and medical schools, there is now a mood of apathy, of defeatism and of excessive material concerns. Clearly, it is time to reverse this national tendency. It will bode poorly for the future of our society and our standing in the world community if this indifferent attitude be allowed to persist.

In our Bicentennial Year we should renew the humanitarian and idealistic thrust that once characterized our national life. In my first State of the State message I noted that "the one resource we must never stint to spend is the well of our compassion for the plight of our fellows. Money may often be short, but imagination, effort and love will be in constant supply." We should review our role in world affairs, and we must give serious thought to re-fashioning our diplomatic priorities. As people dedicated to world peace, we need to recognize the clear and persistent danger to that peace in the existing and widening gap between the rich and the poor, the advantaged and the oppressed, the developed and the still-developing nations of the world. A people poorly fed, poorly cared for, and without hope is a people ready to lash out at enemies, real or imagined, foreign or domestic. I believe that there is no greater threat to world peace today than a series of nations frustrated, embittered and angered by their lack of a safe and secure life. What better way for us to commemorate our Bicentennial Year than to embark on a program to help the less fortunate parts of the world to at least a minimal standard of good health?

The question will be raised, of course, of why we should burden our resources by engaging in foreign health assistance at this time, when our own domestic needs remain unmet and our illusions about policing the world are fast disappearing? The answer can be given on several different levels. First, on a moral level, it is necessary to revive and regenerate the spirit of idealism that gave birth to our nation and so indelibly marked its greatness. Simply because other superpowers act for crass or material purposes, there is no need for us to live down to their standards. Although humanitarian impulses are frequently regarded as sentimental, there is no need for us to deny the spirit of good will and cooperation that should motivate our diplomacy.

On a second level, it can be argued that American statecraft requires new methods in our dealings with the Third World. We can no longer rely upon the simple formulae of industrial assistance, capital investment and the building of new institutions in Africa or on the slopes of the Andes. Millions of the world's people are not impressed by expensive hydroelectric projects or by nuclear reactor programs. Their needs must be met at the grass roots level. They must be met by programs that have an impact on the daily lives and the strength of each family, village, or urban barrio. Too often, Americans in the developing world have not communicated with the starving peasants, the drought victims and the war refugees. They have been largely concerned with the commercial establishment and the military elite. In doing so, they have failed to make the human contact or to deliver the practical benefits that were within our nation's power. There is a need for us to renew our capability to do good and to do it effectively. The establishment of an international medical corps program could provide a modest first step towards meeting the human needs of the Third World.

The third level on which such a program would be beneficial is that of American medicine itself. There are many programs and delivery services that we must develop in our society. There is much that we must attend to in our inner cities, in Appalachia and in Puerto Rico in the areas of improved deployment of community health services, the construction of early warning systems to epidemics, the training of paramedical personnel, and the provision of less expensive hospital care. We need to develop better health systems that will utilize the sub-professional assistant technicians, that will lower drug prices, expand mass immunization, and improve medical surveillance systems in our schools. It is timely and realistic to argue that United States medical programs could be usefully stimulated, enhanced and diversified by proposals that are designed largely for deployment overseas.

Finally, purely from the viewpoint of our national self-interest, important practical benefits can accrue from our altruistic activities abroad designed to relieve human misery. The disparity between the rich countries and the poor countries has grown sharply as a result of the escalation of oil, feed and fertilizer prices. We cannot expect to accelerate our own economic growth and to acquire ever greater industrial power in a world beset with crop failures, vitamin deficiencies, epidemic diseases and mass misery. We cannot expect to recover our national strength solely by curbing inflation at home, by balancing our payments overseas, and by reducing our energy consumption. Nor can we expect to regain our national prestige by retreating into a "fortress America" psychology, ignoring the very real human needs of a large percentage of the world's people.

Clearly then, the United States would benefit both idealistically and pragmatically from providing health assistance to countries that need it. At this particular time in our history, as we begin the third century from our nation's founding, we must look beyond empty rhetoric. We must rejuvenate the sense of generosity that has exemplified our history. We are a pragmatic people who believe in implementing our ideals. Here is a made-to-order situation in which we can demonstrate to the entire world—as well as to our own citizens—that America can manufacture medicines, not munitions, that we can train medical aides, not military experts, and that we can export assistance, not tools of oppression.

Leadership today is a high-risk profession. When you are the one to make the decisions, you discover there are no "right" answers, only an endless array of less than perfect possibilities. There can be no honor in having to close down hospitals. There can be no glory in having to choose who will do without. But tomorrow will come, whatever we wish. And someone is going to shape it, for good or ill. It is the obligation of leaders to determine the priorities of government, to rise above the parochial, to risk the assaults of the greedy and of vested interests in order to fashion a better society. I have openly—and often—cited health care as the top priority in my administration.

Good health is not only a primary goal of both state and national development; it is also an essential means for development through its positive effect on productivity. How can the United States best offer assistance in improvement of health for the people of the developing nations?

There are three types of assistance that the U.S. can offer: 1) ideas and techniques, 2) materials and machines, and 3) consultants, teachers, and workers. How can these types of assistance be conveyed most effectively to the less developed countries.

Ideas and techniques may include: systems for more extensive use of auxiliary health personnel; regionalization; newer techniques for vaccine production, for packaging of medications, rehabilitative procedures, etc. Ideas can be conveyed to colleagues in journals and books, the spoken word of U.S. consultants, and through teaching in either institutional or informal settings.

It is essential to recognize, however, that ideas or techniques originating in the U.S. and other developed countries must be carefully evaluated before use in the less developed countries. Many innovations would be not only inappropriate but harmful, if applied in the wrong social and economic settings.

Material aid should include commodities that can be produced more economically in the United States than in the recipient country—for example, certain pharmaceuticals and vaccines. In offering commodities to other countries, however, we must bear in mind the possibility of stifling potential industries that might provide employment for the citizens of the recipient countries. Recent examples in Iraq and Egypt show the potential for development of the drug industry in providing employment and saving precious foreign exchange.

The third type of aid that the U.S. could offer—personnel—is the most difficult form of technical assistance to plan for, implement and evaluate. The cost of U.S. experts differs from the cost of local health workers in recipient developing countries by many orders of magnitude. While a U.S. jeep may cost somewhat more than a Japanese or locally produced jeep; the cost of U.S. physician consultants, including requisite back-up services, may be more than ten times the cost of a local physician. Furthermore, consultation in international health is a difficult art and success is hard to predict. These difficulties do not mean that the U.S. should go out of the technical assistance consultant business—far from it. They simply emphasize the need for careful planning of the form that our assistance in health to developing countries should take.

Foreign health assistance programs must always take cognizance of the need for nations to assume fuller responsibility for their own destinies. Foreign assistance is often given with the implicit understanding that the donor "knows best" and should determine the forms of aid. Recipient nations have the limited options of accepting or refusing the aid. A new mode of technical cooperation must be developed which will give recipient nations far greater options for "calling the shots." Foreign aid programs should not be a vehicle primarily for employment of U.S. health personnel, for financing of U.S. health training institutions, or for underwriting U.S. pharmaceutical and chemical industry exports. A mechanism should be used whereby recipient nation institutions propose projects and determine the optimum mix of inputs of commodities, training, and consultants. An example of such a program is the International Development Research Centre in Canada.*

*IDRC is a Canadian Crown Corporation, founded in 1970 by an act of Parliament. Although the funds are Canadian the board is international, 10 from Canada and 10 from other countries. The Center's basic purpose is to initiate, encourage and support research into problems of the developing regions throughout the world. The major innovation of the IDRC is that once a decision has been made to finance a project, the direct management is in the hands of developing country partners alone. IDRC reserves only the right for audit and periodic review. The founders of IDRC feel that this style

The U.S. would do well to examine the IDRC and see how its operating principles might be modified to fit our own technical assistance programs.

Given the constraints of the aid that the U.S. can provide, what are the health needs of recipient countries? In a recent paper Lee Howard, the Medical Director of the Agency for International Development, carefully analyzed the issues and identified three key health problems of less developed nations.

INADEQUATE LOW-COST RURAL HEALTH SYSTEMS

Since it is neither feasible nor desirable for the United States to export sufficient high cost medical services and equipment to impoverished countries, we must aid in the development of innovative programs that emphasize delivering medical services economically. Although the United States lacks extensive experience in the training, utilization, and evaluation of physician-extenders, our efforts with nurse-practitioners and physician-associates will give legitimacy to the concept.

Emphasis upon low cost effective delivery systems is imperative. In some countries of the Third World there is suspicion that American technical assistance will promote a hospital-based medical elite and infrastructure whose costs overtax resources. Judging from our past activities, this suspicion is justified, and our image must be changed.

INADEQUATE HEALTH PLANNING

The burden of preventable disease and excessive childbearing is far greater in less developed countries than in the U.S. Lack of health planning in these countries has led to distortion of priorities, putting intensive care units ahead of immunization and family planning. Poor manpower planning has led to the brain-drain of physicians and nurses—expensively trained professionals that poor countries can ill-afford to lose. Poor planning leads to unstaffed hospitals, clinics without medicine, and countless other problems. Although the U.S. does not have great expertise in national health planning, program planning is well-developed, and our experience should be shared with the developing countries.

of international operation removes the stigma of charity and donor control. By 1974 the program had grown to approximately 15 million dollars, the bulk of which was invested in health, population, agriculture and other research programs throughout the world.

MALNUTRITION SECONDARY TO PARASITISM AND INFECTION

It is estimated that there are great losses in food energy from malabsorption due to parasitism and infection, and metabolic losses from fever. Research and application of methods of parasite and infection control are indicated. Other key problems could be identified but we would still be left with the essential question of how to secure the optimum match of our vast U.S. resources with the key needs of less developed countries.

Today, international health is at a crossroads; the old programs and the old techniques are no longer adequate. This is the time for a fresh look at international health problems and resources. This is the time for a group of health experts, from the U.S. and abroad, from Congress and the Executive Branches of Government, to meet and redefine our international health policy.

A Task Force or Commission is often a device to postpone action; in this case, it would be a mechanism to plan action. Ideally, such a commission should, obviously, be formed on the Federal level. I would enthusiastically welcome that. If not so arranged, however, I would recognize my obligation to convene such a critical national and international meeting. New York State houses the United Nations, is the capital of both the business and diplomatic communities, and has long been the refuge of the world.

When a member of the House of Representatives, I introduced a bill in the U.S. Congress to create a pilot program that would have coordinated and supported the multiple governmental and private American medical programs overseas. It would also have committed the United States to identify with a humane program as at least a balance to our military and commercial presence in the developing world. The International Health Agency Act of 1971 gathered support in both the House of Representatives and the Senate, but died in committee because of the opposition of the Nixon Administration. Considering the new mood prevailing in the Congress and in American society, I believe it is time to consider again measures whose benefits could be of great consequence to the soul of this nation as well as to the body of the developing world.

If a U.S. International Health Program is to succeed, it must be closely coordinated with the World Health Organization, the Pan-American Health Organization, with other voluntary agencies, and with appropriate units of both the Department of Health, Education and Welfare and the Department of State. We must not add to inflationary pressures by duplicating bureaucratic structures or overhead costs, but neither should it be supposed that existing agencies can handle a fraction of the work that needs to be done. The World Health Organization and existing U.S. International Health Programs have budgets that are absurdly small in comparison to our G.N.P. of $1.5 trillion a year. For example, the total budget of the World Health Organization is less than *one-tenth* that of the health budget of New York City alone. Indeed, if we spent only 1 percent of our defense and international security expenditures, or .01 percent of our G.N.P., on an international medical project, we would enhance our security as well as our self-esteem. We would also make an immense contribution to the quality of life of millions who are our neighbors in the global village which this planet has become.

Development is far more difficult than sending a man to the moon—and far more worthwhile. It is a challenge worthy of our best efforts.

Thirty years ago, in his Fourth Inaugural Address, President Franklin Roosevelt said: "We have learned that we cannot live alone, at peace; that our own well-being is dependent on the well-being of other nations, far away. We have learned that we must live as men, not as ostriches. . . . We have learned to be citizens of the world, members of the human community." Those lessons were learned in the throes of global war. Let us now put them to work for the retention of global tranquility. Let us understand that the basic rights of life, liberty and the pursuit of happiness, promised in our own Declaration of Independence, mean nothing unless there is protection from disease and disaster. And let us take the first step towards seeking for our fellow men and women throughout the world the most fundamental of all rights: the highest possible standard of health.

IMPACT OF INDEPENDENCE AND NATIONALISM ON TROPICAL MEDICINE

W. Russell Lumsden, D.Sc., M.B., F.R.C.P.E., F.R.S.E.

Professor, Department of Medical Protozoology
London School of Hygiene and Tropical Medicine
London, England

I shall confine my main attention in discussing the impact of independence and nationalism on tropical medicine to the field with which I am most familiar—the epidemiology of those communicable diseases of man and animals which are important in impeding development in the warm countries of the world.

As background for this paper, I shall first mention the experiences which have led to my being asked by Professor Kevin M. Cahill to contribute to this symposium among so distinguished a group of speakers. As a schoolboy and student in the 1920s and 1930s I grew up in the Kipling-influenced environment of the British Empire, in which it was regarded as a duty to devote one's skills to the assistance of one's less fortunate tropical brethren. My original interest in zoology led quickly to an interest in zoology as related to tropical medicine. I was encouraged in this inclination by the manifestly clearer rationale in the study of tropical as compared with temperate-climate disease. In the days before the sulphonamides and penicillin, as a student I was impressed with the apparent certainty with which, for instance, we could cure malaria with quinine as a specific highly effective drug or control the disease with our clear knowledge of its mechanism of transmission. These apparent clarities contrasted with the obscurities of much temperate-climate medicine: for example, the causation of rheumatic heart disease, the uncertainties in the prognosis of lobar pneumonia, and the lack of efficient drugs, and the protracted treatment of such common conditions as sycosis barbae and syphilis.

Five years in the malarial field laboratories in His Majesty's Forces in the Mediterranean and India during World War II altered my convictions regarding the ease with which malaria might be combatted—notwithstanding our drugs and knowledge—even in a young, healthy population under discipline. I remember one evening in North Palestine when the consultant malariologist for the Middle East—the then to me legendary figure Brigadier J. L. Sinton, V. C.—came into our mess enraged about the lack of discipline among troops on the lines of communication to Damascus. They were still in their short trousers late in the evening. This may seem a triviality, but later, in Sicily and in Italy, such lapses were to result in heavy casualties.

After the war I spent 10 years with the Yellow Fever Research Institute, later the East African Virus Research Institute, at Entebbe, Uganda. This institute was at first concerned only with yellow fever; work was directed toward defining its epidemiology in East Africa in human, animal, and insect hosts so as to assess the menace it offered to the areas still unaffected: the Middle and the Far East. Although the basic concept of the epidemiology of yellow fever was important for human health, at this time actual contacts with the effects of the disease were few. Yellow fever was widely distributed in monkeys in East Africa, but rarely caused human infection. Interest transferred later to other arboviral diseases, particularly chikungunya, which, on its first recorded appearance, affected some 80% of the 200,000 members of the Makonde tribe in Newala District, Tanganyika.

Arboviral diseases, although their epidemiology was fascinating—involving, besides man, a wide range of forest and savannah mammals and insects in extremely complicated interrelations—turned out to be comparatively minor impediments to development. Nowadays yellow fever rarely impinges on the human population, and when it does it can be effectively counteracted by an efficient vaccine. Most other arboviruses, such as chikungunya and dengue, may produce epidemics with a high morbidity but these are usually of short duration and low mortality. For instance, the chikungunya epidemic mentioned above affected most of the population with a short-term, acute and painful disease, but caused almost no mortality and affected the general pattern of human existence hardly at all.

I was to be impressed later with the altogether more significant impact upon the human condition of some protozoal and helminthic diseases: malaria, trypanosomiasis, and schistosomiasis. Nevertheless, these early studies of the epidemiology of yellow fever and other arboviruses were of paramount importance for tropical epidemiology and set the pattern for the epidemiological investigation of communicable tropical disease in general.

In 1957 I transferred from the arboviral field to the East African Trypanosomiasis Research Organization (EATRO), into a situation with a quite different degree of urgency. Trypanosome infection in man —sleeping sickness—offered a much greater menace. Sleeping sickness quite literally could extinguish the human occupants of an area; we are not immune to that outcome even today. Trypanosome diseases in domestic animals—nagana—have just as important an effect on cattle. They exclude cattle from huge areas of subsaharan Africa, which are estimated in total to exceed the area of the United States. Over this vast area this is the main reason for the shortage of protein in human diets.

Because of these evident and urgent effects, research in trypanosomiasis—far more than arboviral research—attracted comment and argument from the wide range of different interests that were involved daily with trypanosomiasis as an important and ever-present problem: medical men, veterinarians, farmers, tsetse-control workers, politicians, sociologists, and so on. In this situation it was not always easy to maintain research programs, however essential and likely to be productive they might be in the long term, in the face of demands for "useful" short-term investigations.

Since 1963, when I returned to academic appointments in Edinburgh and London, I have attempted to develop research related to the trypanosome diseases of man and animals in Africa. I have paid particular attention to areas in which it was difficult to progress under the somewhat restricted scientific scope of the East African territories at that time and which may be more profitably followed in the more diverse scientific environment of the United Kingdom.

History of Research Development in East Africa
before Independence

Research in tropical diseases in East Africa began when commissions of scientists were sent out by the Royal Society to investigate the cause of the epidemics of sleeping sickness which devastated most of the circumference of Lake Victoria in the first few years of this century. Some mighty names were involved: Sir David Bruce, Aldo Castellani, David Nabarro, and Muriel Robertson in Uganda, and in Tanganyika, then a

German colonial territory, Robert Koch. These were small groups of workers or single individuals, devoted to narrowly specific investigations: to discover the causative agents of sleeping sickness or nagana and to define their methods of transmission. These scientists laid the foundations of our knowledge of insect-borne disease in East Africa and provided the beginning of systematic scientific research there. A great debt is owed to them, although their relations with one another cannot be said always to have been edifying.[1] Following this early work, a great deal of well balanced research, taking into account many aspects of trypanosomiasis, continued until the 1920s. Then emphasis shifted to a concentration on one aspect only: control of trypanosome diseases by control of the vector *Glossina* (tsetse fly). The decision to concentrate on this aspect appears to have been attributable mainly to the influence of C. F. M. Swynnerton and was based upon the lack of efficient drugs for treatment or prophylaxis, disappointing results from studies of immunity and tolerance to infection, and restriction of the scope of interest in this disease associated with the withdrawal of German workers from Tanganyika after World War I.

This concentration of research on one aspect of trypanosomiasis continued almost unbroken in East Africa until the mid-1950s. Then a return took place to a more comprehensive approach designed to encourage and integrate the contributions of several different scientific disciplines. This broader approach was caused partly by disappointment in the progress gained by concentration on the ecology of the vector, partly by the advent of residual insecticides and of efficient drugs both for cure and prophylaxis, but perhaps even more by a general widening of scientific capability and range of thought in East Africa. The last factor was determined by the growth of a wide range of research institutes and the consequent contacts among their workers. Individual territories were not without their contribution to this scientific change; for example, the Division of Insect-Borne Diseases of the Kenya Government at Nairobi was always an important contributor. However, the main research contribution was made by the interterritorial units.

The first interterritorial unit was the Yellow Fever Research Institute at Entebbe, Uganda, which was set up by the Rockefeller Foundation in 1936. This institute contributed importantly before and during World War II; it was phased over to British auspices in the several years following the war. At this time, a number of research organizations were also developed under the Colonial Development and Welfare Acts, each designed for a fairly specific purpose. Besides the expansion of the Yellow Fever Research Institute to cover viral diseases in general, institutes were set up for malaria, trypanosomiasis, medical survey, and leprosy on the medical side and for crop, veterinary, forestry, and fisheries industries on the agricultural side. At that time these institutes were staffed, of necessity, almost entirely by expatriate scientists, mainly from the United Kingdom, but with some from continental Europe.

As an example of these institutes, I shall discuss the Yellow Fever Research Institute. Yellow fever in East Africa is a zoonosis, i.e., an infection of animals which may be transmitted to man. The work of the institute was based on field studies in particular ecological environments, including studies of man, of the wild and domestic animals possibly involved in transmission cycles, and of the distribution and behavior of possible vectors—mainly *Aedes* mosquitoes. These studies were closely linked with and supported by laboratory-based studies designed to identify the viral agents isolated or antibodies to them and to study viral behavior in mammalian and insect hosts which the field studies identified as likely to be important epidemiologically. These studies were in turn linked with related studies at the home base of the institute—the Rockefeller Foundation Virus Laboratory in New York—to which problems outside the immediate program of the field institute could be referred for study with the assistance of the fuller resources available in a developed country. This pattern has always seemed to me, since that time, to be the paragon of research interrelations and collaborations. Indeed, it was extremely effective; it led to the working out in detail of the epidemiology of yellow fever in East Africa in little more than 10 years by only a handful of workers.

A contrast was evident to me when I transferred to the East African Trypanosomiasis Research Organization. The first two components were there, the field and the local supporting Trypanosomiasis Research Organization, but there was no formal scientific connection with a research center in the United Kingdom. I believe this was the situation in most British institutes. There were no formally designated affiliated institutions in scientifically highly developed countries to which problems could be referred and which had some commitment to assist in their study when they passed beyond the expertise of the East African institutes. Besides the blockages in the progress of research which occur when such assistance is not easily available, the lack of this link contributed to the instability of the expatriate staff at the time of independence. They did not feel that they had adequate support in their home country. In consequence, a large loss of expatriate scientists from East African institutes took place in the years following independence.

DEVELOPMENTS RELATED TO INDEPENDENCE

The foregoing was roughly the situation in 1962 when I wrote a contribution to *Nature*[2] in which I emphasized the importance of good communications between the three main levels of research—the field, the laboratory in the tropics, and the laboratory in the scientifically highly-developed country—and of the appropriate apportionment of particular aspects of the work among them. The difficulties related to independence are basically the difficulties of maintaining such inter-communication under the political changes which have taken place since that time.

For some years before independence, thought had been given to the need to encourage local participation in the research programs. It was clear that most expatriate workers should soon be replaced by African scientists. The institutes made some contribution to training in this respect, as witness the yearly courses on trypanosomiasis which used to be run by EATRO for medical and veterinary students from Kampala and Nairobi. Some of the students introduced to the subject by these courses subsequently came back to work in research in trypanosomiasis. However, since the main commitment of the institutes was to research, they could hardly make more than a minor contribution to training. It was to the East African universities that we looked for the main supply of trained African scientists; support for their growth was the first priority at that time.

There is one development related to the shift of emphasis from institutes to universities which should be mentioned: the shift of major contributions in research from one to the other. Before 1962 the major contributions to research were from non-teaching research institutes set up specifically for particular studies; the contribution of the universities was comparatively minor. Since then the universities have vastly increased in size and importance and the research institutes have been static or even regressed. While the increasing role of the universities in relation to research has many advantages—such as the extension of scientific contact and the more easy interchangeability of staff within the academic world—the change has, inevitably, also blurred the clear sense of purpose and focus which was an important spur in the old style institutes.

The need for local appointments to the staff of the institutes was at no level more important than at the directorial level. In the case of my own retirement from East Africa, there were those who argued that only an African scientist should be appointed in succession. I believed that if this advice were followed it would be 10 or 15 years before an indigenous appointment could be made and that an African with administrative and medical training and with a good appreciation of the control of trypanosomiasis in the field should be sought. This advice was followed and provided satisfactory stable direction of the organization for some eight or nine years. This allowed sufficient time for a worker basically trained as a scientist to grow into the demands of the position. The organization is now under the direction of a biochemist.

However, the transition period since 1962 has been a difficult one. Although there has often been productive cooperation between teams of local African scientists and expatriate visiting workers from Europe and America, there have been also many upsets and dislocations determined by local political changes. The political instability of countries is at present a main cause of difficulty in attracting scientists to the institutes on a long-term basis and, therefore, in the rapid extension of the techniques available for research in East Africa. Nevertheless the potential of the institutes for collaborative work remains high, as it is usually only a short time after the one group of expatriates fades out before another comes forward.

The same transitional difficulties apply, of course, also to the universities, although to a lesser extent as they are more closely connected with the continuity of the academic world as a whole than are the research institutes. One might have expected, as a repercussion following the end of colonial rule, a reaction against expatriate workers, particularly of the nationality of the former colonial power. In fact, this has occurred rather infrequently although, of course, there have been some episodes; since independence British scientists have worked quite successfully in East Africa in collaboration with the institutes. The East African territories have perhaps also enjoyed their new capability of experimenting with the introduction of expatriate scientists from many other countries. Perhaps the situation is changing again as older jealousies die out, to a more positive requirement expressed by developing territories for assistance in the planning and execution of research. It behooves us, therefore, to consider carefully what administrative structure will be necessary for the fulfilment of these needs in a mutually acceptable, stable, and productive way.

A NEW STRUCTURE

Since independence, the most effective lines of action have been obscured and complicated by manifold political and devlopmental considerations. There have been many conferences and discussion groups: the Conference on Joint Research Schemes and Recruitment held by the Centre for African Studies of the University of Edinburgh in collaboration with the Ministry of Overseas Development,[3] the Symposium on Training in Epidemiology and Management of Parasitic Diseases of the World Health Organization,[4] and the Conference on Medical Education, Research, and Medical Care in Developing Countries organized by the Royal Society of Tropical Medicine and Hygiene and the Wellcome Fund.[5] All these meetings have contributed to the planning of research in tropical medicine and veterinary medicine but the actual development of those plans has been less conspicuous.

What are the main considerations to be satisfied if research is to be organized rapidly and oriented toward the improvement of actual disease situations? I shall begin with some of the requirements for maintaining the impetus of research which I presented to the Conference on Joint Research Schemes and Recruitment in 1965, and comment on and extend them in light of experience since that time.

First, of all the other requirements for research—men, buildings, equipment—the first is paramount; all factors should be considered primarily in light of their influence in attracting and retaining a cadre of high-quality workers. In 1960 this requirement consisted primarily of stemming the loss of experienced expatriate personnel from the research organizations. By 1965 few of these people were left and it became even more difficult to produce a setting which would induce the few remaining expatriate scientists to stay and which would encourage a new flow of scientists from training schools in Africa and Europe. The problem of attracting scientists with special skills from outside of Africa has increased steadily since the end of World War II. Immediately after that war newly demobilized scientists were many and opportunities for research few; in 1965 the range of research opportunity in Europe was enormous and a correspondingly greater effort was needed to attract workers to the study of tropical problems. The problem is even greater today. Although many young British scientists still express an interest in working on tropical problems—partly attracted by their own interest in the subject and partly motivated by the social responsibility so keenly felt by many young graduates today—it is difficult to encourage their interest with the promise of a long-term career.

Although there are many more indigenous scientists available in Africa now than in 1965 it is still important for these scientists to be linked to relevant research outside of Africa in temperate countries as this will inevitably be broader in scope, both academically and technically, than that of tropical African territories for some decades to come. Such linking can be best accomplished by attracting scientists with special skills from these countries to work in Africa.

Second, the administrative framework within which the scientists are to work is of importance. It must be stable and able to offer a lifetime's career to be able to attract and retain scientists of the highest caliber. The considerations which are important in this respect may differ according to whether the scientists are indigenous or expatriates from more developed countries. Taking expatriate workers first, as those most needed initially to develop research and train scientists from the developing countries, the most important considerations appear to be:

1) The framework must be based on international organizations rather than on the national governments of developed countries. Support of the framework by national governments alone is not entirely satisfactory, as the interest of national governments in tropical problems may be precarious, varying according to the political or financial influences. International organizations offer advantages in this respect; they must always include tropical problems in their list of responsibilities, therefore they can be expected to maintain an interest in them and to accept the responsibility for studying them.

2) The plan for the framework must take into account that for scientists from Europe permanent assignments in Africa are presently neither desirable nor possible. Terms of service must be such that interchangeability between staffs of overseas institutions and research centers in temperate countries is not impeded by pension or superannuation

arrangements. The structure also must recognize and accept the changing inclination of individual expatriate staff members to serve overseas.
For instance, research workers with small children are usually contented
and efficient overseas. On the other hand, if a research worker remains
overseas for long periods during his children's secondary education his
family life is frequently disrupted. At this stage he is likely to work
more efficiently if placed at a related research center in his home country. Transfers which take account of these factors do not appear to offer
difficulty on scientific grounds. There will always be sections of the
whole investigation which can be followed more advantageously or even
essentially in the most highly developed academic centers. Indeed, inter-
changes of this sort will be essential for the maintenance of fruitful
collaboration between centers in developing and developed countries.

3) As important as the administrative framework will be the scientific framework, as all concerned will demand to be well connected with
the scientific world at large. Thus, the arrangements must connect research organizations among themselves and also with other centers of
scientific activity: local universities, European centers of research and
teaching, and the appropriate international organizations such as the
World Health Organization and the Food and Agriculture Organization
of the United Nations. Centers of research must be located where they
can relate to African field problems, but they must also be in close contact with universities so as to bring African problems to the notice of
undergraduate and new postgraduate students so as to gain their interest
and provide the needed flow of young workers into the field.

These considerations of administrative framework and scientific communication have been discussed primarily with regard to attracting
scientists to Africa to help with African problems, but similar considerations also apply to indigenous African scientists. The best of these scientists will only be attracted to work on these problems if they can look
forward to stable careers which offer a breadth of international accom-
plishments comparable with that enjoyed by workers in developed
countries.

4) Just as important as the organization of research is its orientation,
to ensure that it is channelled into avenues most likely to ameliorate
existing disease situations. In my discussion of this in 1962 I divided
research in East Africa into two types: type A—specifically and narrowly limited to the practical problem in question: type B—still directed

toward the solution of practical problems, but in which the approaches likely to be successful were undefined. It is in this second type that the doctrine of good communication is most important. The avoidance of isolation, the appropriate location of research, and the planning of research groups of optimum size are some of the important factors in securing good communication, which will ensure the continual reappraisal of plans and ideas so that research is most advantageously orientated toward the solution of problems of immediate practical importance.

In 1965 I drew attention to the need for planning comprehensive studies specifically directed to the elimination of some of the blockages in our present knowledge which keep us from a full understanding of the epidemiology of sleeping sickness. An example is the need for methods to differentiate between man-infecting strains of *Trypanosoma brucei* from those which do not infect man; this is an essential prerequisite for understanding the epidemiology of the disease. Advances have been made in both immunological and biochemical characterization and in other methods of differentiation such as by sensitivity to human serum. But attention has been only desultory and a concerted attack on the problem has not materialized.

A parallel example, which has come to my attention since I came to London, is the recognition of infection with *Trypanosoma cruzi*, the organism responsible for Chagas' disease in South America. The most widely used method for diagnosis is xenodiagnosis, which consists of allowing laboratory-bred insects to feed on suspect cases and examining these insects microscopically for organisms for up to 90 days subsequently. The presence of organisms in these insects indicates the presence of disease in the suspected case. Such a method of diagnosis is almost grotesquely unattractive and inefficient. First, it involves the exposure of the patient to these distasteful insects. Second, the diagnosis may be delayed as much as three months. Third, the examination of these insects introduces a serious hazard of infection to the workers who dissect them since they may be carrying highly infective organisms of a kind against which no really effective chemotherapy is yet available. There is a need for a concerted attempt to produce better methods.

There are multiple examples of problems of this kind which require specially planned, concentrated, and comprehensive studies for their solution. There is need for a mechanism to agree upon the problems of greatest urgency and to assign a task force to study them, perhaps by assembling a research team more comprehensive than is available at any individual research center. This would be feasible if the resources of all African and European centers of research could be drawn upon. International collaboration would be required for the planning of such studies; the international organizations would seem to be the appropriate bodies to arrange such cooperation.

CONCLUSION

I have been able merely to touch upon a few of the principles which I consider most important to maintain the impetus of research in tropical medicine in directions which will be likely to lead to an improvement in the field situations within a reasonable time. They are presented *in vacuo*, with little regard to the multiple political, social, and personal problems which would have to be overcome for their systematic development. In 1965 I commented that, although the international organizations seemed to be the natural base for comprehensive studies of this sort, since the proposals for a World Health Research Center had had to be shelved, the only course seemed to be to make use of national arrangements and to interrelate the several national contributions as closely as possible through international organizations.

This comment related to a proposal by Dr. M. G. Candau, then secretary-general of the World Health Organization, to set up a World Health Research Center to be concerned with three main objectives: 1) epidemiological, for the study of the world distribution of disease, 2) communications, for the processing of information, and 3) biomedical matters. Debate on that proposal in the British press and medical journals between January 1964 and December 1967 on the part of the proponents was concerned mainly with the value of such an organization to the world as a whole and in particular with the suitability of Edinburgh as a location. Opponents were concerned with the fears of established research organizations that such a foundation would draw off their best workers. I was not convinced by the latter argument. Although good workers may transfer to other organizations if the opportunities for carrying on their research are better, this cannot but have a good and stimulating effect, in that it increases the competition in the field of research and so the likely rate of progress.

Looking back on the correspondence on that debate from nearly 10 years later, one is impressed with the slowness of progress on blockage problems as compared with what might have been accomplished had a center been established. In the outcome, the "scattered [research] groups" advocated by Swann in place of the research center[6] have contributed much of interest, but much more could have been accomplished by a concentrated and orientated approach, so that by now advances could be applied in the field. The whole debate is well summarized and put into proportion by Lord Ritchie-Calder,[7] who pointed out that the gaps found in the more random method of support for research stimulated the Medical Research Council of the United Kingdom to set up the National Institute for Medical Research (NIMR). He compared the proposed research center to the NIMR on an international scale.

Today the need for a coordinating and integrating center continues to make itself felt; it has resurfaced recently in the proposal for a central, multidisciplinary, coordinating and research institute for advanced training and research in the biomedical sciences to be established at Ndola, Zambia.[8] In the light of previous experience, this proposal is to be commended, but perhaps it should be considered whether some part of the institute should not be in Europe, as previously proposed, so as to form a link which would ensure the interest of developed countries in subjects of tropical importance and draw upon their expertise—which will remain more comprehensive than tropical expertise for some decades to come. Financing such developments will be a problem at the present time; perhaps the international organizations might assume the role of negotiators to stimulate and integrate contributions from the widest possible range of sources, including national governments, philanthropic foundations, and international development funds.

REFERENCES

1. Lumsden, W. H. R.: Some episodes in the history of African trypanosomiasis. *Proc. Roy. Soc. Med.* 67: 789-96, 1974.
2. Lumsden, W. H. R.: The organization and orientation of research in underdeveloped areas. *Nature* (London) 195:1139-41, 1962.
3. *Conference on Joint Research Schemes and Recruitment.* University of Edinburgh, Centre of African Studies (in association with U.K. Ministry of Overseas Development), 1965.
4. *Symposium on Training in Epidemiology and Management of Parasitic Diseases.* Geneva, WHO, 1971.
5. Commentary on a conference. Royal Society of Tropical Medicine and Hygiene and Wellcome Fund. *Trans. Roy. Soc. Trop. Med. Hyg.* 65, 709-721, 1971.
6. Swann, M: Inside story of the WHO Centre. *The Scotsman,* December 19, 1967.
7. Ritchie-Calder, The Right Hon. The Lord: Who did what to WHO? *The Scotsman,* December 23, 1967.
8. *Special WHO Programme for Research and Training in the Developing Countries on Parasitic and other Major Communicable Diseases.* Geneva, WHO, 1974.

WORLD HEALTH:
AN ETHICAL-ECONOMIC PERSPECTIVE

THE RIGHT HON. THE LORD RITCHIE-CALDER, C.B.E.

Center for Democratic Studies
Santa Barbara, Calif.

THERE is a Scandinavian proverb: "The little birds would not sing so sweetly if they knew how poor they are." It is a nice thought which at least distinguishes between being poor and being miserable, but it does not explain that hungry birds do not sing and that sick birds curl up and die.

When the world is too much with us and good intentions go astray we (and I include myself) are tempted to say "Why interfere? Why not let them be?" And then I remember a yaws-ridden Arcadia in Java.

Practically the entire population of a district in the Javanese hills had yaws. The *Spirochaeta* of yaws enters the body through cuts and sores; where people work barefoot in the fields it is easy to get cuts and to contract the disease by contagion. It afflicted all age groups, from the baby with the fly-blistered mouth sucking at its mother's breast to the old people—although old was a relative term; the expectation of life of a new-born child in that region was less than 30 years. The disease shows itself in ugly sores but it also pervades the body, enters the bones, and eats away the soft tissues. It destroys the spirit of the people because the hopelessness of the disease leaves them nothing for which to live. The disease can scar a landscape as surely as it disfigures bodies: We could recognize a region of yaws by the neglected fields, the neglected cattle, the neglected children, and the neglected homes.

Before World War II the Javanese doctors had tried to fight the disease with arsenicals. After the war penicillin was available; for the price of an ice-cream sundae, a glass of beer, or a few cigarettes a human life could be transformed. With penicillin the World Health Organisation (WHO), together with the United Nations Children Fund (UNICEF) and a dedicated Indonesian public health service, as part of the worldwide yaws campaign launched an attack in the hills of central Java.

I was with a team which visited a remote hill village. The people were summoned to receive their penicillin shots by the beating of gongs made from hollowed tree trunks. It was a grim sight. Living skeletons were carried in palanquins. Many came crippled and crawling with the claw-foot which occurs when yaws enters the sole and makes the foot contract like the claw of a perching bird.

One little boy who came crawling was called Tresno; I made friends with him and held him when he got his injection. Ten days later we reassembled for the checkup and that little boy—who in his young life had never had reason to smile—came running and smiling up the path to greet me.

A year later I heard from a friend in that region. He wrote:

> You remember the day that Tresno smiled? That was exactly twelve months ago. Today was a feast day—celebrating the disappearance of yaws. Since that day a year ago, children have been born into a life without yaws. Youngsters had almost forgotten what it was but grown-ups remembered and they had a feast. Everybody contributed. Tresno climbed palm-trees to collect coconuts. Men brought fish and rice which they had been able to harvest without yaws. The women plucked chickens. The headman beat the gong and the children came chattering and laughing, skipping and jumping. The *gamelin* band beat out the tunes and old and young joined in the dancing—the dancing they had almost forgotten. People boasted about the size of the ulcers they once had. The local "comic" put on an act, imitating the walk of the claw-footed yaws' victims and everybody roared with laughter—the gusty laughter of a remembered nightmare. The men teamed up in a dumb-show in which they mimed the painful slow-motion harvesting of the rice when they had yaws and worked up with the tempo of the *gamelan* band to the prodigies of speed with which they could now reap. And Tresno's smile had turned to laughter.

I do not know how you express that in a cost-benefit ratio, but no money could buy for me the satisfaction I feel from knowing that I was there to help the little birds to sing.

Let us look at Central Java and the chain of events which flowed from medical intervention. The WHO/UNICEF teams did a dramatic job there in the control of yaws and malaria.

In the Hungry Hills, as we called them 20 years ago, the people's diet had been coconuts, bananas, and cassava. They looked down on the paddy fields of the plains, but to them rice was a luxury. They wanted to grow rice, but this requires large amounts of water and the Progo River bypassed their slopes. With their liberation from debilitating diseases they took the initiative and began to cut a canal from the headwaters of the Progo along the volcanic ridge in order that they could have steep-tiered terraces, flushed by cascades of water from above.

The sight was unforgettable. In the crude cofferdam which was holding back the headwaters they were digging and delving in the mud and scurrying like ants up swaying bamboo ladders with baskets of rubble on their heads. Along the line of the canal, whenever they encountered rock they would chip it to pieces with hammers and chisels. They had no gelignite—only their muscles and primitive tools. This was the way the Hillah Canal must have been made to carry the waters of the Euphrates around Babylon; but these were not slaves; they were freemen working on voluntary levees. Work which mechanical shovels or bulldozers and a few sticks of explosives could have accomplished in days took them months. In a year they had progressed only two and one half miles.

As we stood in the equatorial sun watching them I became more and more indignant. This was the 20th century, not the days of Babylonian bondage! When an irrigation expert from the United Nations who was with me remarked, "Isn't it a wonderful sight?" I protested. I said I was going straight back to Djakarta to demand the equipment they ought to have.

"Don't you dare!" he replied. "Try to understand. This is *their* canal. For the first time they will have something they don't owe to the money-lenders. Always they have been in debt for the means of their own existence. If anyone offers them material help at this stage, they would never believe it was disinterested. They would think it was another device of the money-lenders. Let them get on with it in their own way and when they have accomplished their purpose, we can help them in other ways."

Experience since then has proved to me that he was right. Most of our mistakes in aid projects have been made because we (the patronizing *we*) believed that we knew what they *needed* and never considered what they *wanted*—when *we* did things for them and not with them. But look at it another way: if we had given them that equipment they would have had the food which they desperately needed much quicker. There was a choice, but the Javanese made the choice.

Ten years later I went back to central Java. Before World War II central Java had been a rice bowl, exporting rice to other parts of Asia. Throughout the region the peasants, like those working on the Progo canal, had been industrious and responsive to new ideas (when they were fit). They had created the paddies of the valley floor and the living pyramids of rice-growing terraces. After the war they had listened to the advice of their agricultural extension services and foreign experts. They had learned the virtues of green manure, better seeds from the state seed farms, and better management of irrigation. They had improved their aquaculture and the traditional methods of growing fish with their rice. When the fields were flooded and the rice planted they introduced *Tilapia* fingerlings from the state fish farms. The fingerlings flourished in the flooded fields; when the fields were drained to harvest the rice the fish would be about the size of pilchards and could be harvested at the same time. The production of food in central Java had increased by 2.5% a year.

However, after this industrious 10 years, conditions of chronic famine existed for much of the population. I call this chronic famine because in the Congo and elsewhere I have seen some of the worst forms of acute famine when, by appealing to the compassion of the world, we had rushed in relief. In Java I saw the prevalence of marasmus, the walking skeletons; nutritional edema; kwashiorkor, the children with rusted hair and skins cracked like a crazy paving; xerophthalmia, the blindness of vitamin deficiency; and infants dehydrated by hunger. The medical services had established day-and-night clinics to treat these diseases.

Why? Because, while the production of food had increased by 25% in 10 years, the population had increased by 30%. That 5% difference meant hunger in all its gradations from malnutrition to starvation.

This illustrates the ethical-economic dilemma. A. V. Hill, winner of the Nobel Prize for medicine, posed the problem in his presidential address to the British Association for the Advancement of Science in 1952:

> Had it been possible to foresee the enormous success of the application of medicine and hygiene would humane people have agreed it could better have been held back, to keep in step with other parallel progress? Some might say "yes" taking the purely biological view that if people bred like rabbits they must be allowed to die like rabbits, until gradually improving education and the demand for a higher standard of life teach them better. But suppose it was certain now that the pressure of increasing population, uncontrolled by disease, would lead not only to the exhaustion of soil and other capital resources but also to the continuing and increasing international tension and disorder, making it harder for civilization to survive, would the majority of humane people change their minds? If ethical principles deny our right to do evil in order that good may come, are we justified in doing good when the foreseeable consequence is evil?

As I said at the time, the ruthless logic to be derived from A. V. Hill's rabbit analogy would be to invent a human myxomatosis. "We" would kill "them" off like pests battening on "our" civilization, wasting "our" soil and squandering "our" capital resources. But who are we and who are they? As Rudyard Kipling said in *Debits and Credits:*

> Father and mother and me,
> Sister and auntie say,
> All good people like us are "we"
> And everyone else is "they"
> We live over the way
> While they live over the sea
> But—would you believe it!
> "They" look upon "we"
> As another sort of "they."

"We" presumably are those who decide what happens to other people. But if you attend the United Nations General Assembly you would find that we and they have got rather mixed up. It would seem that the "we" role has been assumed by the Arab oil-producing states, which are largely underpopulated. Recently I attended the United Nations *Law of the Sea Conference* in Caracas, Venezuela (June-

August 1974), where the "we"—who were calling the cards—were the less developed coastal states of Latin America, Asia, and Africa. And at the United Nations *Population Conference* in Bucharest (November 1974) the voices of what had been A. V. Hill's "they" were articulate in their reluctance to face the facts of population increase which are worse than they were when A. V. Hill expressed his anxieties.

Twenty years ago, when I spoke of the food and population problem I would say "Every time the clock ticks, there is another mouth to be fed." Today I say "Every time your pulse beats there are three more mouths to be fed," or, more melodramatically, "Every day the equivalent of 20 divisions of Martians invade this planet without their field rations."

Let us consider the medical responsibility for this. At a symposium held in Stockholm recently by the Nobel Foundation to consider the human predicament, an economic historian suggested that the so-called population explosion in what we now call "underdeveloped" and once called "backward" countries began at the beginning of the 20th century when the advanced countries, with the spreading of their empires, started to transfer their health practices to their colonies. That was a slow process, which does not adequately explain the present size of populations. The acceleration of this trend can be explained as the result of the direct intervention of medical science and pharmaceutical technology.

We can cite the exact second of the first nuclear explosion on July 16, 1945 in the desert of Alamogordo. We cannot be that precise about the population explosion, but I would say that the fuse was set 10 years earlier in February 1935, when a desperate father injected a red dye into his daughter who was dying of generalized septicemia. She survived. The father was Gerhard Domagk and the red dye was the sulphanilamide, prontosil, the first of the sulpha drugs. It is symbolic that the first extensive use of prontosil took place in Queen Charlotte's Maternity Hospital, London, where it arrested an outbreak of puerperal fever. It saved the lives of those mothers so that they could bear more children.

The sulpha drugs demonstrated that it was possible to kill specific germs within a living body without killing the host at the same time. This made it possible for Howard W. Florey and Ernst B. Chain to look back in 1938 at Alexander Fleming's discovery of penicillin in

1928, and recognize (as he admitted he had not) that it could be used to inhibit germs within the living body. The discovery of dichlorodiphenyltrichoroethane (DDT) in Switzerland at the outbreak of World War II provided the insecticide against the vectors of disease. These three—the sulphas, the antibiotics, and the antivectors—were given war-time priorities in production; the results were remarkable. The infections and contagions, which throughout all the wars of history had killed more than military weapons, were contained.

At the end of the war stockpiles of the drugs and the potential for mass production were available to stem the epidemics expected in the war-ravaged countries, with broken armies and displaced persons on the move. The United Nations Relief and Rehabilitation Agency (UNRRA) distributed the drugs in the refugee camps and through the public health services of countries staggering back to normalcy. Again the results were convincing. In Cyprus and Sardinia the first effective control of malaria was achieved within a short time.

The benefits of the new armory of pharmaceuticals were extended to the tropical countries. UNICEF inherited from UNRRA (when it was disbanded ungraciously and prematurely) the responsibility for the world's children. When the WHO came into existence in 1948 they formed a partnership, with UNICEF acting as the supply agency and the WHO providing the professional staff and advice. The same relation was established between UNICEF and the Food and Agricultural Organization (FAO) and the United Nations Scientific and Cultural Organization (UNESCO). The WHO also inherited a vigorous campaign using bacillus Calmethe-Guérin (BCG) from the Scandinavians, which had been successful in restraining tuberculosis in war-ravaged countries.

And thereby hangs a cautionary tale. BCG is, of course, a prophylactic against tuberculosis which was easy to mount with Mantoux tests and vaccine. I remember going around India with a BCG team. When we arrived in a village a summons would go out, a procession would be organized, and the people would join in and march to the mobile clinics. The drill would be gone through and people would get their injections. But simple-minded people (including politicians) do not distinguish between prophylaxis and treatment. Here, so it seemed, was the answer to tuberculosis.

Tuberculosis became a political issue. Governments insisted that the WHO should help them to set up clinics for active cases of tuberculosis. Against its better judgement, the WHO helped to conduct surveys and open clinics in India, Burma, and other countries. It provided international experts to instruct local doctors, nurses, and paramedical auxiliary personnel and it helped to provide equipment such as x-ray machines. The results were embarrassing to all concerned. Diagnosis was easy enough, but how to treat the cases that were diagnosed? In India the first superficial findings showed that a minimum of three million beds in sanatoria would be needed at once. In Rangoon, when the clinic was opened people lined up, 300 a day were examined, and thousands were turned away—people from every walk and condition of life. For there were no hospital beds and no sanatoria; all that could be done had to be on an outpatient basis. Active cases were sent home to overcrowded conditions. Health visitors would make visits, mainly to exhort and teach these people how not to infect others; little could then be done for the ambulatory cases themselves.

What dismayed members of the WHO was the fact that some governments regarded the mere gesture of opening clinics as a pretext for ignoring the conditions which produced tuberculosis—poor housing, inadequate nutrition, poor sanitation, and so on—as a slovenly housewife sweeps the dust under the carpet. If the results of poverty could be treated, poverty itself did not matter so much. The governments did not and could not provide the hospitals necessary for treatment.

The WHO's embarrassment was qualified by the development of anti-tuberculosis drugs such as streptomycin with para-aminosalycilic acid (PAS) which made it possible to treat outpatients. But it was "back to the drawing board" in public health practice because the clinical elements were subject to local conditions and could not be generalized from one set of circumstances or locality to another. There have been refinements of the drugs and redefinition of the practices, but the inescapable fact which the directors-general of the WHO, Brock Chisholm and Marcallino Candau, realized was that tuberculosis is still a disease transmitted by poverty and that pharmaceuticals are merely palliative.

Let us take other examples of the ethical-economic perspective, to which I shall add the political dimension. A social and political chain reaction can be started with a glass of milk.

When Afghanistan became a member of the United Nations its ambitions in terms of technical assistance were modest: it called in UNICEF to provide dried milk for its children. Dried milk was then available to UNICEF at nominal prices because of surpluses in the United States, and milk depots could readily be established for Afghan children. But, whither UNICEF goes thither goes the WHO. Alongside the milk depots mother-and-child health clinics were established by the WHO and staffed—as was necessary in a Mohammedan country—by female pediatricians, gynecologists, and obstetricians since no male doctor could examine a woman in purdah. A masterful stroke was accomplished when the UN agencies persuaded the daughters—royal princesses—of the prime minister and cousins of the king to become trainees in midwifery.

The purdah women, veiled from head to foot in the all-concealing *shardris,* would bring their children for a supply of milk and would find themselves in a clinic where—sanctioned by the presence of the princesses—for the first time they met professional women, unashamedly unveiled, educated, honored, and respected as women. So the hidden woman began to learn that women were important and that she in turn was important—not just as a breeding machine or as a chattel—and that she deserved and should get the best medical attention. From a glass of milk, a social revolution began—the emancipation of the hidden woman.

I was there 10 years later when the king issued a proclamation allowing women to unveil and I remember the daughters of Afghan friends—young girls whom I had met but never seen—greeting me with barefaced exultation and telling me how they had taken not only their own *shardris* but those of their protesting mothers and had burned them in bonfires. Immediately they claimed their places in the University of Kabul so that soon 25% of the undergraduates were women—women studying civil engineering, nuclear physics, electronic engineering, and, appropriately, considering the origins of it all, medicine. Things have changed in Afghanistan. The adventurous king has been deposed without violence, but his efforts for the emancipation of women has not been undone.

Let us look at another socioeconomic chain reaction. After independence the government of India decided to recover for food production the jungle in Uttar Pradesh—the locale of Kipling's jungle books.

This was a malaria-ridden area of 2,000 square miles. It was a product of over-ambitious technology 800 years ago, when an energetic peasantry cut lateral canals between the tributaries of the Ganges. Unfortunately, canals were cut across the natural drainage and the area became a swamp. The swamp bred malaria-bearing mosquitoes which killed or drove out most of the population, turning the land over to Shere Khan (the tiger), Kaa (the python), and Bandar-log (the monkey) of the jungle books. The king of that jungle however was Ping, the mosquito, who held rich arable land in fief.

To recover the land, the WHO first had to get rid of the mosquito. The international team under a distinguished Greek malariologist, Peter Issaris, moved in with all the usual paraphernalia of trucks and spray-guns, but they ran into immediate difficulties. The jungle region was sparsely inhabited by two tribes: the Tharus and the Bhuksas. In lore, and perhaps in actual history, they were strange tribes. According to their traditions a princely house of the Rajputs had gone to war and all the royal males had been killed. The princesses had escaped into the jungle with men of two of the servant subcastes, the Saises and the Chamars, and their offspring were the Tharus and Bhuksas, respectively. But since the female founders had been princesses, the females of the tribe, reversing the usual pattern in India, remained the dominant sex. (Students of Kipling will remember Kim and the woman of Shamlegh, who dominated her male harem. Shamlegh is in this region.)

The tribes were truculent; they refused to cooperate and closed their villages to the spray teams. This was not unnatural, since no one had entered this jungle in the past except for hostile reasons and all those trucks and spray-guns were not reassuring. After all, mosquitoes are tiny things.

Then the English public health nurse mounted an elephant with her tiger gun and set off for the villages, as did her Indian counterpart in a sari. The nurse did not offer arguments; she just sat around until a child with an infected eye came along (all local children had infected eyes). Then the nurse would put on some of her *khol* or mascara (made of carbon-black and ghee, a rendered butter, was smeared by the tribal mothers on their children's eyes not as a cosmetic but as a treatment). Then the nurse would go away and return a week or so later. There would be a line of children with sore eyes waiting for her because the mothers had realized that her *khol* was really effective—as it should

be, since it contained chemotherapeutics. Soon the women would discuss their own ailments with her and shortly she was on intimate and
friendly terms with them. Within a few weeks it was the women, persuaded by a woman, who threw open the villages and the huts to the
men with the insecticides.

When I traveled that jungle with her, I asked the nurse how she
managed this without knowing the language or, at that time, the tradition of female domination of the tribe. Proving that people are much
the same the world over and that medicine is a craft as well as a science,
she explained that she had been a district nurse in England, where one
of her jobs had been to persuade proud old country people to go to a
hospital when they believed that they were going to the workhouse.
"When you can persuade old people to go to the hospital when they
think it is the workhouse, the Tharus and the Bhuksas were no problem
at all," she said.

Malaria was eradicated and the FAO moved in to clear the jungle
with bulldozers, tree-dozers, and ploughs. Tube wells were installed so
that irrigation could be provided with ground water and the water table
was lowered so that the topsoil no longer was saturated. Refugees from
the Pakistani Punjab were brought in and have farmed it well.

In these and other instances the social sequellae are important. As
countries have discovered when inviting international agencies, the initial
project—staffed by international experts, financed and equipped by
the agencies, and employing native workers to be trained to take over—
is often the least of it. The control of malaria is accompanied by requirements of public health and clinical medicine, which include follow-up
reinforcements by fully qualified professional and paramedical personnel. There is an immediate need for clinics, hospitals, and general practitioners, and then there is a need for more schools. When malaria is
prevalent, perhaps two thirds of the children registered may be absent
on any given day, but when malaria is controlled all will be in attend-
ance. Both accommodations and teachers have to be found—classrooms
for elementary education, secondary schools to provide the cadres for
higher education, centers for paraprofessional training, universities, and
medical schools.

In addition, of course, there is a concomitant increase in population
to be considered. The population explosion is not the result of a great
orgy of procreation. Couples are not having more children than they

once did (although we might hope they would have less). Mothers such as the women saved by prontosil in Queen Charlotte's Hospital are surviving the hazards of childbirth and living to have more children. Children are surviving the infections of infancy and childhood to marry and multiply. Adults in the developing countries are living longer, although the span of life is still far short of the life-expectancy in richer countries. For example, the life expectancy of a girl born in India in 1948 was 27 years; today it is 48 years. This means that the average woman will live through her reproductive lifespan and can continue having children who will have an increased expectation of survival. A couple, once dependent on children for manual labor in the fields or for security in old age, would have had 14 or 15 children, with the expectation that four or five would survive; now most children survive.

Public health, medical science, and pharmaceutical technology have cut off the peaks of the curves of the old mass-killer diseases. The result is that at this moment more than half the children in the less-developed world are less than 15 years of age. The prediction that the population will be doubled by 2000 A.D. is almost a biological certainty. The young will mate and have children; even with the most intensive and extensive birth-control campaign, world population will reach not less than seven billion. Without birth-control measures it could be more.

I am energetically involved in promoting family planning but ultimately two people must make their own decision. No amount of exhortation about the demographic or economic consequences will ultimately persuade them. They must be convinced, informed, and provided with the means for birth control, but with the freedom to make the final decision as to how many children they want. If the medical profession, the public authorities, and the other life-saving agencies of the world could convincingly say "We keep children alive," couples would limit the size of their families.

I assume that all of us agree, while we might want fewer children to be conceived, that any child who is born is entitled to survive and that our health-care services (with all due respect to A. V. Hill) must be deployed to that end. We have, in the enlightened phrase which came out of the United Nations, to "invest in human resources." We have to use the same ingenuity which medical science has used to change the patterns of disease to take the imperative measures which will provide for the material needs of the present and future population of the world. The knowledge exists and could be called upon. What is lacking is the political will.

We have never adequately financed, equipped, or morally supported the UN agencies to which we ostensibly have given this responsibility. As Professor Kevin M. Cahill has pointed out, the total budget of the WHO allocated for the health needs of the whole world is one tenth that allocated for health and sanitary services in New York City. We blunder into crises and then pass the responsibility to the international organizations which we have starved of sufficient funds. Or we improvise costly emergency operations without considering their side effects.

The problem of food and population is not new. As has the poor, it has always been with us because it is another side of poverty. There is no inherent difference—except the scale of unpreparedness—between the situation which is scaring us now and what was obvious a quarter of a century ago. Both Brock Chisholm, the first director-general of the WHO, and Boyd Orr, the first director-general of the FAO, recognized the cycle of misery, the carousel of calamity: endemic disease, underproduction, squalor, ignorance, malnutrition, more disease. People who are sick cannot produce food nor earn the means to buy it. If they are hungry they will have no aptitude for learning. If they are ignorant they cannot better themselves. They are reduced to squalor; they are malnourished and vulnerable to disease. They succumb to the old litany of hunger: better to walk than to run; better to sit than to walk; better to sleep than to sit; better to die than to sleep.

Where countries are poor, human resources are turned from living assets into social liabilities. When we were promoting the National Health Service in Britain our slogan was "The health of a country is the wealth of a country." This is true of the whole world. There is no "we" and "they"—just "we" in a world which has shrunk to a neighbourhood.

THE ECOLOGY OF DISEASE
IN THE TROPICS

HERBERT M. GILLES, M.D., F.R.C.P.

Alfred Jones-Warrington Yorke Professor of Tropical Medicine
University of Liverpool

Professor of Tropical Medicine
Liverpool School of Tropical Medicine

Liverpool, England

MOST tropical countries are faced with many problems of com-
munity-wide endemic and sometimes epidemic diseases which
may have disastrous physical and economic effects on the population.
As a background to these diseases there are nutritional, environmental,
socioeconomic, and genetic factors which affect the people directly or
influence the progress of the disease patterns themselves.

"Third World" countries cannot achieve healthy economies without
considerable permanent improvement in the health of their people.
Therefore, there are impelling human and economic reasons for acceler-
ating the study of prevalent diseases and morbid states with a view to
their control and possible eradication, with a consequent improvement
in standards of living. Whether one is dealing with disease in urban or
rural areas of the tropics, the outstanding obstacle to a rational approach
to the control of disease is the relative lack of valid statistical data on
population and its distribution, birth rates, death rates, and the incidence
of disease in terms of mortality and morbidity. Before any plan for the
control of disease in Africa, for example, can be soundly formulated, we
must secure substantial data on the actual incidence and morbidity of
disease in both rural and urban areas by establishing appropriate studies.

The Akufo Village scheme, the results of which have already been
published,[1] was designed to focus attention on the community and to
stress the importance in its medical pattern of the interplay between
diet, environment, and social and genetic background in a rural population in Western Nigeria. The philosophy behind the scheme, however,
is equally applicable to other rural areas of the tropics.

Age in years

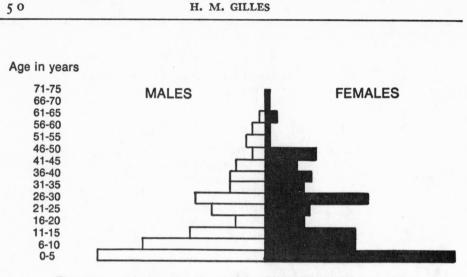

Fig. 1. Age and sex pyramid of a typical tropical rural population.

An important development in the tropics is the relatively recent establishment of large dams aimed at providing hydroelectric power and expanding agricultural potential through large-scale immigration. These socioeconomic development schemes, however, give rise to health problems which cannot be ignored.

DEMOGRAPHY

In many areas of the tropics young persons less than 14 years of age make up more than 40% of the population, in marked contrast to the situation in the developed countries of the world. Examination of the age and sex pyramid of tropical rural populations (Figure 1) reveals the following striking features: 1) a broad base reflecting a high fertility rate and a high wastage of child life, 2) a relative absence of adolescents as a result of migration to the cities, 3) a preponderance of women between the ages of 20 and 39 resulting from the polygamous habits of men in some countries, and 4) a small number of persons more than 60 years of age. This demographic pattern is fairly widespread throughout the rural tropics but, as might be expected, it is not universal and important variations occur, especially in urban areas or as a result of differing social, cultural, and religious habits. The incidence of twinning is extremely high in some areas of the tropics—especially in Nigeria, Taiwan, and Egypt.

In the more developed countries the population pyramid shows a gradual decline, indicating the relatively older population with a low death rate in childhood. In practical terms it is still the problems of maternal and pediatric care that concern us in the tropics, in contrast to those of geriatric care and noncommunicale disease in the developed world.

CHILDHOOD MORTALITY

Great caution must be exercised in accepting and interpreting death rates in the tropics. However, most observers would agree that, although discrepancies occur not only between village and village but also from year to year, childhood mortality in many areas of the tropics is still very high. The improvement of health services has undoubtedly already lowered these mortalities in many areas, but there are still remote rural areas where the situation has not materially improved. In any case, it is a salutary thought that the mortality of children under five years of age that I recorded at Akufo over the four-year period 1959-1962 was of the order of population; this was within 12 miles of the modern teaching hospital at Ibadan. In 1973 the childhood mortality (less than five years of age) recorded by a village scribe in a small rural village of Nigeria was 38%.

AGRICULTURE

Since the economies of many tropical countries are still basically agricultural and the largest proportion of their populations still live in rural areas, land use has a direct bearing on the economic life and dietary patterns of tropical communities. The data on the percentage of cultivated land under each crop in a typical West African village is illustrated in Figure 2. Differing land-use patterns will naturally be found in areas where groundnut or palm-kernel grows; where cotton or jute is the main cash crop; and where rice, plantain, sweet potatoes, or red beans are the staple diet.

NUTRITION

In large areas of the tropics malnutrition, especially in young children, is one of the principal causes of morbidity and mortality. The problem of feeding the populations of the world and thereby maintaining an adequate level of nutritional health is a serious one. Its magnitude and severity have only recently received attention; there has been

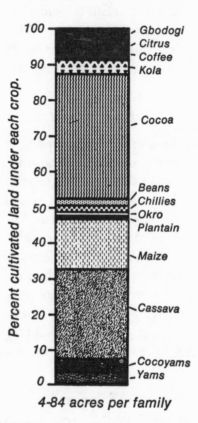

Fig. 2. Cropping pattern at Akufo, A Nigerian Village.

no completely reliable assessment in quantitative terms. Hunger, as manifest through famines or chronic undernutrition, has been recognized from prehistoric times. However, the problems related to the absence of specific nutrients have begun to be understood only relatively recently.

Human malnutrition is an ecological problem; the following intimately related factors may be involved in its pathogenesis: 1) production and distribution of food, 2) storage and processing of food, 3) demographical problems related to food (the rate of increase of the population in most developing countries is more than 2% and the rate of increase of food production in most areas has not kept up with the population increase), 4) education and sociocultural factors, 5) the preparation and consumption of food, and 6) the role of infection.[2]

Some agencies of the United Nations have estimated that about one

third of the world's population goes to bed hungry every day—mostly
in the countries of Asia, Africa, and Latin America. The most vulnerable
groups are infants, preschool children, and pregnant and nursing mothers. Protein-calorie malnutrition is the name accepted now for a disease
syndrome which includes kwashiorkor, believed to be largely caused by
a deficiency of protein, and nutritional marasmus, which is caused by a
general deficiency of all nutrients, especially calories. In tropical communities one sees cases ranging from one extreme to the other. Among
adults acute periods of undernutrition may occur in large populations
because of the failure of food crops or catastrophes of one kind or
another: floods, earthquakes, wars, and a lack of rain.

The background of conditions of nutritional deficiency is extensive
and can be seen to be more dependent on the socioeconomic level of the
society than almost any other disease. Lack of sufficient protein and
calories is the world's most important nutritional problem, although
deficiencies of vitamin A, B, and D are also quite common.

It has become more and more evident that the interaction of nutrition and infection are so intimate that it is absurd to attempt to dissociate
the two factors; it is obvious that only an integrated approach to both
problems can meet with success. For example, the general nutritional
status of young children in the rural villages of the plateau of Nigeria
is good, with mean serum albumin levels of 3.6 g $\pm$ 0.7 gm./100 ml., yet
childhood mortality remained abnormally high because of the heavy
load of infection borne during these early years.[3]

COMMUNICABLE DISEASES

Communicable diseases are widespread in the tropics and occur at a
much earlier age than in Europe and America. They are particularly
prevalent and an important cause of morbidity and mortality in the
preschool child.

In India tuberculosis still kills half a million people a year and there
are more than 5 million cases; cholera and smallpox are major problems;
there are 2.6 million cases of leprosy. Other diseases such as trachoma,
diphtheria, poliomyelitis, rabies, and hemorrhagic fever are common.[4]
Measles is endemic in many areas; in West Africa it is considered one
of the most fatal diseases of the preschool child.[5, 6] Pneumonia and
bronchopneumonia, tetanus, whooping cough, and other infections are
rampant.

Diarrheal diseases also represent a major public health problem in many developing countries. Although widespread in the tropics, they most severely affect the preschool child—the critical period being one to four years of age. Some of the acute diarrheas are specific infective diseases: e.g., shigellosis and salmonellosis; another major portion have no demonstrable infectious agent. The death rates from diarrheal diseases are impressive in themselves. In three Guatamalan villages over a 10-year period they ranged from 12 to 36% in children less than five years of age, with a maximal mortality in the second year of life.[7] For school children and adults the rates are a fraction of those in the earlier years of life. Disease-specific rates of mortality have been found to be higher in poor than in richer countries by the following factors: influenza, pneumonia, and bronchitis, 2.3; respiratory tuberculosis, 5; dysentery (all forms), 7.5; typhoid fever, 160; diphtheria, 100; whooping cough, 300; and measles, 55.[8]

PARASITIC INFECTIONS

Polyparasitism is extremely common; as many as nine species of parasites may cohabit in the same host. In both rural and many urban environments the water used for drinking, washing, and other domestic purposes is a source of guinea-worm and schistosomiasis. The food eaten, both meat and vegetables, is a source of tapeworm, roundworm, and whipworm. Where fresh-water fish or crustacea are consumed liver or lung flukes predominate. The soil transmits hookworm and stronglyoidiasis, while the profusion of biting insects convey malaria, trypanosomiasis, onchocerciasis, or filariasis. Dogs, cats, and other animals in the houses and yards predispose humans to zoonotic parasitic infections such as toxocariasis and assist the mechanical spread of intestinal helminths.

Malaria still assails some 500 million people and causes about one million deaths annually. Some 300 million persons live in contact with schistosomiasis, 250 million with filariasis, and 20 million with onchocerciasis (associated with river blindness). Trypanosomal infections threaten 50 million Africans and a similar number of South Americans (in Brazil Chagas' disease accounts for a third of all adult deaths). Leishmaniasis affects some 7 million persons, while the number of persons exposed to (and probably infected by) intestinal helminths such as hookworm is thought to exceed 1,000 million.[9]

Noninfective Diseases

Important noninfective diseases, e.g., endomyocardial fibrosis, add to the complexity of the environment, and some malignant conditions, e.g., primary liver-cell carcinoma, Burkitt's tumor, and choriocarcinoma, although cosmopolitan, predominate in tropical countries. In many tropical countries coronary artery disease is still rare, but in others it is becoming increasingly common.

Genetics

Interest in genetics has been greatly stimulated in the tropics and subtropics by the discovery that high gene frequencies for some genetic traits are maintained by providing a protection to the carrier against falciparum malaria.[10] The genetic markers vary in importance from one area to the other. Thus, while hemoglobin S is the most important abnormal hemoglobin in Africa, it is superseded by hemoglobin E and thalassemia in Southeast Asia. In Africa sickle-cell anemia has an incidence of nearly 2% in some countries and may be responsible for a childhood mortality of approximately five deaths per 1,000 population.

Social Factors

Social factors may also play an important role in the genesis of disease in the tropics. Thus in New Guinea "enteritis necroticans"—a diffuse sloughing enteritis of the intestines—is related to pig-feasting, which is an integral and complex part of the indigenous culture of all highland tribes. Similarly, the changing epidemiology of the fascinating disease kuru is associated with the fact that cannibalism has been abandoned among the Fore tribe with the penetration of western civilisation to the hinterlands of New Guinea.

Urbanization and Industralisation

One of the most significant changes taking place in the tropics is the migration of people from rural to urban areas where industrial and commercial enterprises are developing. The proximity of slums and shanty towns to modern buildings and large department stores commonly occurs. In Singapore, for example, the medical problems are no longer those of communicable disease but of multistory apartments and population pressure. Very little is known yet of the sociomedical implication of living in high-rise apartments, especially in a multiracial society such as Singapore, in which momentous changes in mores and attitudes are occurring.

So far, the reductions in population growth achieved by family planning have been small and reasonable success has been attained only in a few of the smaller and more highly developed areas with advancing industrialization, high literacy rates, good standards of living and education, and good health services. These include Singapore, Hong Kong, and Taiwan in particular. In the larger and slower-developing countries, especially India, attempts to mount family-planning programs have had mixed results and on the whole have not been highly successful.

SOCIOECONOMIC DEVELOPMENT

Man has converted for agriculture and hydroelectric power vast inhospitable and unproductive areas of Africa, the Middle East, and Southeast Asia by water conservation or the harnessing of rivers. If such schemes are to be fully productive, health care must be included as part of the general planning at all stages, for the health of a population can have enormous economic and social implications.

Schistosomiasis, for example, has been spread in the Sudan by the Gezira water-development scheme and in Ghana by the Volta Dam. Indeed, in Ghana, what is almost an epidemic of *S. haematobium* infection has occurred among the settlers around the lake. *Truncatus rohlfsi*, a snail known in the area for years but never hitherto able to act as an intermediate host for schistosomiasis in Ghana, has, under the new ecological conditions created by the lake, become the predominant intermediate snail vector.

In Thailand, since the Ubolratana Dam was finished in 1968 the prevalence of opisthorchiasis has been increasing in the population in the immediate vicinity of the new lake as a result of the infection of fish seeded into it for the provision of protein. A different breed of fish (not of the cyprinoid family) would have provided the protein without the opisthorchiasis. A special human feature of the building of the Ubolratana Dam has been the resettlement of the people who had lived and worked in the newly flooded valleys of the small Pong and Choen rivers. In some areas the resettled villagers have been forced to adapt to an entirely new kind of life; the traditional growing of rice has been replaced by the cultivation of cash crops such as jute, with the crudely-milled rice of river villages replaced by the finely-milled and vitamin-

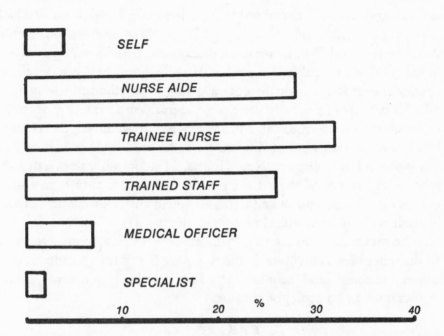

Fig. 3. Health-personnel requirements of the population of a fishing village in New Guinea.

deficient grain of the market towns. Similar social and health problems of resettled populations have occurred at Wadi Halfa in the Sudan following the flooding of the area by the Aswan Dam.

Health Manpower

It is impossible to dissociate the problems of health manpower in the tropics from medical education and the ecology of disease. In the developing countries many medical schools are still producing the "basic" curative doctor by patterns of teaching which, more often than not, have been transposed almost *in toto* from some curricula in Europe or the United States. Such training is satisfactory for practice in cities and towns where the necessary facilities exist. This training is essentially curative; it produces a doctor who is conditioned to deal with sick individuals who are often hospitalized, but it is not designed for practice in fringe urban or rural areas where 80% or more of the population may live and where the major national health problems exist.

A satisfactory health service for a country in which the population is largely rural can be operated only on the basis of a health team in which doctors are trained to function together with nonprofessionals who share the responsibility. In addition, doctors must be trained to function in the existing national health service. If the national health service is to operate successfully, with the doctor acting most efficiently in concert with his colleagues on the health team, the problem of training doctors—the problem of the medical curriculum—is not so much determining how many as what kind of doctors are to be produced. In a three-year study of a fishing village in New Guinea, Maddocks[11] has evaluated the relative importance of the various members of a medical team in a small community. In his improvised clinic he found that most ailments could be dealt with by nonmedical personnel (Figure 3).

The prevention and control of disease are inextricably involved with all the other factors involved in the way men live, with agriculture, education, planning, and economics.[12] The practicing physician in the tropics must be an ecologist at heart.

REFERENCES

1. Gilles, H. M.: *Akufo: An Environmental Study of a Nigerian Village Community.* Ibadan, Ibadan University Press, 1965.
2. Sai, F. T.: The Epidemiology and Control of Nutritional Diseases. In: *A Short Textbook of Preventive Medicine for the Tropics,* Lucas, A. O. and Gilles, H. M., editors. London, English Universities Press, 1973, p. 240.
3. Collis, W. R. F., Dema, I., and Omololu, A.: On the ecology of child health and nutrition in Nigerian villages. I. Environment, population and resources. *Trop. Geogr. Med. 14:*140, 1962.
4. Pattanayak, S., Singha, P., and Arosa, D. D.: Problems of communicable diseases. *First Southeast Asian Regional Seminar Trop. Med.* Bangkok, SEAMES, 1967, p. 61.
5. Morley, D., Woodland, M., and Martin, W. J.: Measles in Nigerian children. A study of the disease in West Africa, and its manifestations in England and

other countries during different epochs. *J. Hyg.* (Cam.) *61:*115, 1963.
6. Hendrickse, R. G. and Sherman, P. M.: Morbidity and mortality from measles in childhood seen at U.C.H. Ibadan. *Arch. Ges. Virusforsch. 16:*27, 1965.
7. Gordon, J. E., Behar, M., and Scrimshaw, N. S.: Acute diarrhoeal disease in less developed countries. 1. An epidemiological basis for control. *Bull. WHO 31:*1, 1964.
8. Cockburn, W. C. and Assaad, F.: Some observations on the communicable diseases as public health problems. *Bull. WHO 49:*1, 1973.
9. Editorial. Immunology and developing countries. *Lancet 2:*632, 1974.
10. Allison, A. C.: Protection afforded by sickle-cell trait against subtertian malarial infection. *Brit. Med. J. 1:*290, 1954.
11. Maddocks, I.: Personal communication, 1974.
12. Maegraith, B. G.: *One World.* London, Athlone, 1973.

THE RELEVANCE OF RESEARCH IN TROPICAL MEDICINE TODAY

JOSEPH H. BURCHENAL, M.D.

Director of Clinical Investigation
Field Coordinator, Human Cancer
Memorial Sloan Kettering Cancer Center
New York, N.Y.

WHEN I was asked to discuss "The Relevance of Research in Tropical Medicine Today," I was instructed in inverted paraphrase of President John F. Kennedy's famous quotation to: Ask not what we can do for research in tropical medicine but rather ask what research in tropical medicine can do for us. In other words, what are the spinoffs of research in tropical medicine? By spinoffs I do not mean the treatment of the occasional traveler who comes home with malaria, leishmaniasis, trypanosomiasis, or dysentery, the treatment of military personnel in the tropics, or the occasional small outbreak in the United States when military personnel carry back a tropical disease. Rather, I shall illustrate how research in tropical medicine or, more broadly, research on disease in the tropics has benefited the treatment of disease here at home.

There are many roadblocks in research. It was Charles Kettering, the inventor of the self-starter on automobiles and of the two-cycle diesel locomotive engine who believed that many discoveries are delayed because of the erroneous notion that they are impossible.[1] The importance of research in tropical medicine has been and still is to demonstrate by analogy the possibilities in the developed countries of some lines of research heretofore considered impossible and to suggest unthought of areas of investigation.

Since my field is cancer I shall concentrate mainly, although not entirely, on the benefits that have accrued in this area. First, let us compare the distribution of tropical disease and cancer in Africa. Trypanosomiasis and malaria have peculiar distributions according to the ecology of their vectors, the tsetse fly and the mosquito. This peculiar distribution has pointed up the vectors responsible and helped in the eradication of these diseases. The population of Africa, at least until recently, has been relatively stable and for that reason studies on the distribution of cancer have been extremely valuable. For instance, hepatocellular cancer of the liver has an extremely high incidence in some areas and is rare in others. So, too, carcinoma of the esophagus is epidemic in certain villages and almost unheard of in others close by. The drinking and eating habits of the people in these particular areas of high and low incidence of cancer are under study. It may well be that potential causative factors such as aflatoxin in liver cancer can be eradicated from the American as well as the African environment, and thus help to prevent hepatocellular carcinoma in this country.

One of the most important African tumors in terms of its contribution to this end is Burkitt's tumor.[2] The peculiar distribution of Burkitt's tumor,[3] which is similar to malaria in that it does not occur at the equator above 5,000 feet, in Rhodesia above 3,000 feet, or in South Africa above 1,500 feet, indicates dependence on climate and suggests that there may be an insect vector.[4] A virus known as the Epstein-Barr (EB) virus has been found to be associated with cultures of Burkitt's tumor for the past 10 years.[5] Patients with the tumor have high titers of antibodies against the virus but significant titers also occur in many normal individuals in that area of Africa and even in the United States. Further research on Burkitt's tumor and the EB virus demonstrated purely by accident that high titers of antibodies to this virus were also present in patients with infectious mononucleosis and that only patients who previously had no antibodies to the virus contracted infectious mononucleosis.[6] Thus, this EB virus, which is present in Burkitt's tumor, and appears, but as yet has not been proved, to have an etiologic role in that disease, has been demonstrated to be the cause of infectious mononucleosis in the United States. These data lead us to ask why primary exposure to this virus in the United States causes subclinical disease in young children but in young adults it can cause infectious mononucelosis, whereas in Africa it usually causes no clinical disease but may be associated with Burkitt's tumor in patients who live in areas with a high incidence of malaria. In this regard, Burkitt's recent studies in Kinshasa and Zanzibar suggest that in areas that have been cleared of malaria there is a very low incidence of Burkitt's tumor, but that when malaria returns so, too, does Burkitt's tumor.[7]

In Africa, carcinoma of the lung and colon, the two biggest killers in the United States, are extremely rare. The low incidence of pulmonary cancer is presumed to be connected with the rarity of cigarette smoking among Africans (except recently among the westernized Africans in the cities). The low incidence of cancer of the colon may be a result of different dietary and bowel habits among the Africans. Burkitt emphasizes that the average African does not feel that he is well unless he has three bowel movements daily. The large amount of roughage in the African diet leads to the rapid transit of food through the intestine, in contrast to the much more prolonged time required to transport the refined, low-roughage food in the intestine of the American and European. Burkitt postulates that this longer transit gives any potential carcinogen a greater time to work on the intestinal mucosa or allows more opportunity for precursors to be converted by the bacteria in the colon into carcinogenic substances.[8] These illustrations give an indication of what may be learned about the etiology of these tumors from their distribution in Africa and the implications of these findings for improving health in the United States.

Departing for a moment from cancer, we must recognize that other studies also are of great value. We are all particularly interested here in arteriosclerotic heart disease and its high incidence in Americans. Studies done in Kampala have shown that Asians, who in India would be expected to have a low incidence of cardiovascular disease, develop a very high incidence of cardiovascular disease when they come to Africa and reach a higher economic status. This appears to be associated with higher economic status, coupled with more sedentary working habits and an increased consumption of meat and fats.

The Masai, who are nomadic tribesmen, also have a diet high in milk, fat, and cholesterol, but their blood-cholesterol levels are low and there is a relative absence of cardiovascular disease. This may due to genetic differences in the ability to handle saturated fats. More probably it is due to their continuous high level of exertion, especially because of the tremendous distances that they walk each day following their herds. Both of these studies have obvious implications for the prevention of cardiovascular disease in the United States today.

In New Guinea there is a bizarre nervous disease known as kuru[9] which appears to be caused by a peculiar slowly growing virus, presumably transmitted by cannibalism. Obviously cannibalism does not occur in the United States, but because of the discovery of this virus a somewhat similar virus has been demonstrated in Creutzfeldt-Jakob dementia in this country;[10] these studies also may have bearing also on amyotrophic lateral sclerosis and multiple sclerosis. In addition, other slow viruses have been implicated in animal tumors and are being sought in human cancer.

I shall now discuss the relation between the chemotherapy of tropical diseases and the chemotherapy of cancer because here especially we owe a great debt to research in tropical medicine. I suggest that the roots of present-day chemotherapy of cancer lie in the chemotherapy of tropical and infectious disease and began about 1630 with the unknown Jesuit who lived among the Incas of Peru and used a tea made of the bark of the chinchona tree to treat malaria. Following this there was an hiatus of more than 200 years; nothing of importance happened in the field of chemotherapy until the great Paul Ehrlich showed the effects of methylene blue on malaria and the dye Trypan Red on the trypanosomes of nagana, a disease which killed horses and cattle and made large areas of Africa unliveable for livestock. Based on this work on trypanosomes[11] was the more important discovery in 1909 of salvarsan,[12] which was active against the spirochaete of syphilis. This and other closely-allied arsenical derivatives were the only curative chemotherapy for syphilis for the next 30-odd years.

In 1934 Mietsch and Domagk,[13] following Ehrlich's example with parasitic disease and Mietsch's own success in synthesizing Atabrine for malaria, were synthesizing and studying a series of dyes against streptococcal infections of mice. The next year Domagk[14] reported the discovery of the antibacterial activity of the red dye, prontosil, and the conquest of streptococcal disease. This was followed by the discovery that this miraculous activity lay only in a small part of the molecule[15] and the enunciation somewhat later by Woods[16] and Fildes[17] of the theory of antimetabolites. Domagk's discovery of the possibility of chemotherapy of infectious disease allowed the resurrection by Florey and Chain[18] of Fleming's discovery of penicillin[19] which had been buried for 10 years. This led to the great age of the chemotherapy of infectious disease. It also led many of us to believe that the chemotherapy of cancer was possible.

During World War II studies already afoot in the chemotherapy of cancer were leading to useful agents. Now that chemotherapy was considered a possibility, Heilmann and Kendall[20] studying the steroid, compound E, later named cortisone, against advanced lymphosarcoma in mice, demonstrated almost total regression of tumor. From this original work came the use of cortisone [21, 22] and finally prednisone, initially in the acute leukemias and now in many forms of combination cancer chemotherapy.

Work of the group connected with the Chemical Warfare Service on the nitrogen mustards demonstrated that these substances would destroy lymphoid tissue in normal animals and would indeed produce regression in mouse lymphosarcoma and chronic leukemias. The success of the antimalarial program during World War II led to the development of a similar type of screening for drugs used against cancer. From this and the original work on nitrogen mustard have come a host of active derivatives such as chlorambucil and Myleran.[23, 24]

From the demonstration by Woods and Fildes of the metabolite-antimetabolite relation of para-aminobenzoic acid to sulfanilamide came the synthesis of the 4-amino folic acid antagonists. Two of these, aminopterin and methotrexate, are used in the clinical treatment of acute leukemia in children.[25] The same research also stimulated the classic systematic studies of antimetabolites of the purines and pyrimidines by Hitchings, Elion, and their group[26, 27] against parasitic diseases and tumors which led to the synthesis and the clinical use of mercaptopurine and thioguanine.

The discovery of penicillin by Fleming and its development by Chain and Florey ushered in the golden age of the use of antibiotics against infectious disease and also against cancer. Actinomycin-D, which is curative in at least 50% of the cases of choriocarcinoma of the uterus, mitomycin-C, daunomycin, adriamycin, and bleomycin are but a few of the active antibiotics useful in cancer.

With these new drugs appearing on the scene, the treatment of the acute leukemias of childhood gradually improved so that the median survival time increased from less than four to as much as 18 months, but most patients eventually became resistant and died of their disease. The studies of Burkitt, Clifford, and Oettgen[28-30] and their colleagues in Africa in the early 1960s, however, demonstrated that Burkitt's tumor, the most common childhood tumor in Africa, which defied surgery and usually killed in three to four months, could be caused to regress completely by high doses of methotrexate or cyclophosphamide; in approximately 15% of these patients there was no recurrence of the disease. These studies, carried further by Ziegler et al.,[31] have shown that 73% of patients with Stage I and Stage II Burkitt's tumor and 50% of all patients with Burkitt's tumor, including those with far advanced Stage III and Stage IV disease, can be brought into long-term remission by the administration of these drugs. Since none of their patients who remain in their original remission more than 18 months have suffered relapse, these long-term remissions are presumed to be synonomous with cure. This demonstrated the curability of a spontaneous tumor in children and led to cure of the acute leukemias and Hodgkin's disease by means of intensive intermittent combinations of drugs; this has increased the median survival time in childhood leukemia to approximately five years. Since most of these patients are still in their original remission and free of all evidence of disease, it seems likely that a high percentage will remain in remission indefinitely or, in other words, are cured. With similar intensive combination therapy in Stage III and Stage IV Hodgkin's disease, approximately 50% of patients are surviving five years without evidence of disease.

In a protocol which was originally based on Ziegler's work in Africa, Wollner et al.[32, 33] have recently obtained striking results in non-Hodgkin's lymphoma, both in the nodal and extranodal type in children, by means of massive doses of cyclophosphamide, followed immediately by radiation therapy to any localized lesions and a regimen used for the treatment of acute lymphoblastic leukemia. Eighty percent of the patients now show no evidence of disease 15 to 40 months from the start of treatment.

Another African contribution came in the treatment of Hodgkin's disease. In the United States early Hodgkin's disease is ordinarily treated by radiation therapy; this is extremely successful, and chemotherapy is used only for the advanced stages. In most of sub-Saharan Africa, however, no radiation facilities were available. For this reason, in Uganda Ziegler[34] and his group treated Hodgkin's disease with chemotherapy of the type which had been shown in the United States to be useful in 50% of patients with advanced disease. All seven of the patients who were in the early stages of the disease went into remission with chemotherapy alone and none had relapsed at the time of the report.

It is well recognized clinically and experimentally that surgery and radiotherapy are limited not by the bulk of the disease but by its spread, whereas chemotherapy is limited by the mass of the tumor rather than its spread. Thus, it would appear from the clinical studies of Ziegler and the data obtained in animals that chemotherapy is more successful when the burden of tumor is small than when it is large. This consideration led to the use of combined chemotherapy immediately after operation in cancers where the primary tumor could be removed by surgery or radiation but where the recurrence rate and eventual failure from tiny metastases present at the time of surgery was high; examples are Wilms' tumor, Ewing's tumor, and osteogenic sarcoma. Ewing's tumor of bone in children and young adults treated with radiation to the primary tumor alone has a high rate of recurrence; at 24 months less than 10% of the patients are free of the disease. However, with combination chemotherapy started immediately after radiation,[35] 60 to 87% of patients are free of disease and apparently cured 24 months to seven years after treatment.[35, 36] In osteogenic sarcoma the results have been even more surprising. Here is a tumor which has a dismal record with surgery alone, where 50% of the patients have pulmonary metastases within five to nine months after operation, 80% have pulmonary metastases at 18 months, and survival is only 20%. When various types of chemotherapy are used immediately after operation the results are startling. Jaffe and Frei[37] and Cortes et al.[38] report that more than 90% and 77%, respectively, of patients treated with intensive chemotherapy immediately after adequate operation are free of disease six to 24 months after operation. That this represents something more than a delay in the development of pulmonary metastases is suggested by the results of Sutow et al.,[39, 40] who applied similar therapy and reported that 10 of 18 patients showed no evidence of disease from 27 to 41 months after operation and nine to 23 months after the discontinuance of chemotherapy.

More important, however, is the suggestion from these two series that aggressive chemotherapy of a relatively refractory tumor is only palliative when the tumor is large but may be curative when the residual growth is minimal. Thus these studies point the way to more successful treatment of solid tumors in adults. High-risk types of carcinoma of the breast, lung, and colon would seem to be ideal targets for such multidisciplinary therapy.

In my excitement about the results that have been achieved recently in the combined treatment of cancer, I have perhaps strayed from tropi-

cal medicine, but to summarize: Research in tropical medicine has
yielded leads to factors causing degenerative neurologic diseases, coronary disease, and several types of cancer. In addition, studies on the
chemotherapy of tropical diseases have led to the chemotherapy of
infectious disease which has achieved the conquest of most of the
diseases of bacterial and rickettsial origin in this country and, similarly,
has given leads to the chemotherapy of cancer. What has been learned
from treating a few special tumors in Africa has greatly improved the
results of therapy in this country in some cancers and points the way
to much greater advances in the future. Research in tropical medicine
is indeed a two-way street. Although its primary goal is the prevention
and treatment of disease in the developing countries, it has made and
is continuing to make contributions to the health of developed countries.

REFERENCES

1. Burchenal, J. H.: Fifth Annual David A. Karnofsky Lecture. From wild fowl to stalking horse: Alchemy in chemotherapy. *Cancer.* In press.
2. Burkitt, D.: A sarcoma involving the jaws in African children. *Brit. J. Surg. 46*:218-23, 1958.
3. Burkitt, D.: Recent Developments in Geographical Distribution. In: *Treatment of Burkitt's Tumor*, Burchenal, J. H. and Burkitt, D. P., editors. Berlin, Heidelberg, New York, Springer, 1967, p. 36.
4. Williams, M. C.: Implications of the Geographical Distribution of Burkitt's Lymphoma. In: *Treatment of Burkitt's Tumor*, Burchenal, J. H. and Burkitt, D. P., editors. Berlin, Heidelberg, New York, Springer, 1967, p. 42.
5. Epstein, M. A., Achong, B. G., and Barr, Y. M.: Virus particles in cultured lymphoblasts from Burkitt's lymphoma. *Lancet 1*:702-03, 1964.
6. Henle, W. and Henle, G.: The relation between the Epstein-Barr virus and infectious monoculeosis, Burkitt's lymphoma and cancer of the post nasal space. *E. Afr. Med. J. 46*:402, 1969.
7. Burkitt, D. P.: Etiology of Burkitt's lymphoma—An alternative hypothesis to a vectored virus. *J. Nat. Cancer Inst.*

42:19, 1969.
8. Burkitt, D. P.: Possible relationships between bowel cancer and dietary habits. *Proc. Roy. Soc. Med. 64*:964, 1971.
9. Gajdusek, D. C.: Kuru in the New Guinea Highlands. In: *Tropical Neurology*, Spillane, J. D., editor. London, New York, Toronto, Oxford University Press, 1973, pp. 376-83.
10. Roos, R., Gibbs, C. J., Jr., and Gajdusek, D. C.: The clinical characteristics of transmissable Creutzfeldt—Jakob disease. *Brain 96*:1, 1973.
11. Ehrlich, P. and Shiga, K.: Farbentherapeutische Versuche bei Trypanosomernerkrankung. *Berl. Klin. Wschr. 41*:329, 1904.
12. Ehrlich, P. and Hata, S.: *Die Experimentelle Chemotherapie der Spirillosen.* Berlin, Springer, 1910.
13. Domagk, G.: Ein Beitrag zur Chemotherapie der bakteriellen Infektion. *Deutsch. Med. Wschr. 61*:250, 1935.
14. Domagk, G.: Eine neue Klasse von Desinfektionsmitteln. *Deutsch. Med. Wschr. 61*:829, 1935.
15. Tréfouel, J., Tréfouel, J., Nitti, F., and Bovet, D.: Activite du p-aminophenyl-sulfamide sur les infections streptococciques experimentales de la

souris et du lapin. *Compt. Rend. Soc. Biol. 120:*756, 1935.

16. Woods, D. D.: The relation of p-aminobenzoic acid to the mechanism of action of sulfanilamide. *Brit. J. Exp. Path. 21:*74, 1940.

17. Fildes, P.: A rational approach to chemotherapy. *Lancet 1:*955, 1940.

18. Chain, E., Florey, H. W., Gardner, A. D., Heatley, N. G., Jennings, M. A., Orr-Ewing, J., and Sanders, A. G.: Penicillin as a chemotherapeutic agent. *Lancet 2:*226, 1940.

19. Fleming, A.: On the antibacterial action of cultures of a penicillin with special reference to their use in the isolation of B. influenza. *Brit. J. Exp. Path. 10:*226, 1929.

20. Heilman, F. R. and Kendall, E. C.: The influence of 11-dehydro-17-hydroxycorticosterone (Compound E) on the growth of malignant tumor in the mouse. *Endocrinology 34:*416, 1944.

21. Farber, S. et al.: The effect of ACTH in acute leukemia in childhood. In: *Proc. 1st Clinical ACTH Conf.,* Mote, J. R., editor. New York, Blakiston, p. 328.

22. Pearson, O. H. and Eliel, L. P.: Use of pituitary adrenocorticotropic hormone (ACTH) and cortisone in lymphomas and leukemias. *J.A.M.A. 144:*1349, 1950.

23. Galton, D. A. G., Israelis, L. G., Narbarro, J. D. N., and Till, M.: Clinical trials of p-(di-2-chloroethylamino)-Phenylbutyric acid (CB 1348) in malignant lymphoma. *Brit. Med. J. 2:*1172, 1955.

24. Haddow, A. and Timmis, G. M.: Myleran in chronic myeloid leukaemia. Chemical constitution and biological action. *Lancet 264:*207, 1953.

25. Farber, S., Diamond, L. K., Mercer, R. D., Sylvester, R. F., Jr., and Wolff, J. A.: Temporary remissions in acute leukemia in children produced by the folic acid antagonist, 4-aminopteroylglutamic acid (Aminopterin). *New Eng. J. Med. 238:*787, 1948.

26. Hitchings, G. H., Elion, G. B., Falco, E. A., Russell, P. B., and VanderWerff, H.: Studies on the analogs of purines and pyrimidines. *Ann. N.Y. Acad. Sci. 52:*1318, 1950.

27. Hitchings, G. H. and Rhoads, C. P.: 6-Mercaptopurine. *Ann. N.Y. Acad. Sci. 60:*183-507, 1954.

28. Oettgen, H. F., Clifford, P., and Burkitt, D. P.: Malignant lymphoma involving the jaw in African children: Treatment with alkylating agents and Actinomycin-D. *Cancer Chemother. Rep. 28:*25, 1963.

29. Oettgen, H. F., Burkitt, D. P., and Burchenal, J. H.: Malignant lymphoma involving the jaw in African children: Treatment with methotrexate. *Cancer 16:*616, 1963.

30. Burkitt, D. P.: Chemotherapy of jaw tumors. In: *Treatment of Burkitt's Tumor,* Burchenal, J. H. and Burkitt, D. P., editors. Berlin, Heidelberg, New York, Springer, 1967, p. 94.

31. Ziegler, J. L.: Chemotherapy of Burkitt's lymphoma. *Cancer 30:*1534, 1972.

32. Wollner, N., D'Angio, G. J., Burchenal, J. H., Lieberman, P., and Fang, S.: Treatment of non-Hodgkin's lymphoma in children with multiple drug leukemia regimen and radiation therapy. *Proc. Amer. Ass. Cancer Res. 14:*97, 1973.

33. Wollner, N., Lieberman, P., Exelby, P., D'Angio, G. J., Burchenal, J. H., Fang, S., and Murphy, M. L.: Non-Hodgkin's lymphoma in children: Results of treatment with LSA$_2$-L$_2$ protocol. *Proc. 5th Meeting Int. Soc. Pediat. Oncol.* Amsterdam, October 1973; personal communication.

34. Ziegler, J. L., Bluming, A. Z., Fass, L., Magrath, I. T., and Templeton, A. C.: Chemotherapy of childhood Hodgkin's disease in Uganda. *Lancet 2:*679, 1972.

35. Hustu, H. O., Pinkel, D., and Pratt, C. B.: Treatment of clinically localized Ewing's sarcoma with radiotherapy and combination chemotherapy. *Cancer 30:*1522, 1972.

36. Rosen, G. Wollner, N., Wu, S. J., Hadju, S. I., Cham, W., D'Angio, G. J., and Murphy, M. L.: Prolonged disease-free survival in children with Ewing's sarcoma treated with radiation therapy and adjuvant 4-drug se-

quential chemotherapy. *26th Ann. Meeting James Ewing Soc.*, April 1973.

37. Jaffe, N., Frei, E., Traggis, D., and Bishop, Y.: Adjuvant methotrexate and citrovorum-factor treatment of osteogenic sarcoma. *New Eng. J. Med. 291:994*, 1974.

38. Cortes, E. P., Holland, J. F., Wang, J. J., Sinks, L. F., Blom, J., Senn, H., Bank, A., and Glidewell, O.: Amputa-

tion and adriamycin in primary osteogenic sarcoma. *New Eng. J. Med. 291: 998*, 1974.

39. Sutow, W. W., Sullivan, M. P., and Fernbach, D. J.: Adjuvant chemotherapy in primary treatment of osteogenic sarcoma. *Proc. Amer. Ass. Cancer Res. 15:20*, 1974.

40. Sutow, W. W.: Personal communication.

ECONOMICS AND HEALTH

G. A. COSTANZO

Vice Chairman of the Board
Citicorp and First National City Bank
New York, N.Y.

ALTHOUGH separate disciplines, health and economic development have made history together. The widespread introduction of western medicine throughout the developing nations began in the late 18th century with the arrival of colonial administrators, military officers, and especially trading-company managers. Among the arrivals were doctors who were to tend the needs of the colonial party and of a fortunate few of the local populace who held significant positions in the colonial structure. Subsequent increased commercial activity spread western medicine further, but rarely to large segments of the indigenous population.

Folk medicine was already well established in such countries as India by the start of the colonial period. It was not until the second half of the 19th century that colonial administrations began to open local schools which taught western medicine. These new schools rarely flourished. Dependent on support from locally-generated revenues, they had to compete with administrative and police services for funds. Medical care suffered because colonial administrators often were reluctant to assert their authority against local religion and custom. Consequently, both western and indigenous medicine failed to make great headway in most of these countries.

In the 20th century World Wars I and II and the great depression caused further setbacks for medicine. During each of the global events doctors were withdrawn from developing countries to serve the citizens of their home countries.

Since World War II a new effort has been mounted, led by the multinational political and economic organizations and aid programs of the developed countries. Despite a paucity of statistics, information

gathered by the World Health Organization (WHO) and other institutions reveal a monumental task yet to be accomplished in bringing
adequate health care to much of the world. In most countries the
ratio of doctors to population is less than one to 50,000. In parts of
the world 40% of children die before four years of age, a proportion
reached in the United States only at 60 years of age. Per capita expenditure for health care in some countries is less than 40 cents per
year. It is estimated that up to one billion people are hungry or malnourished and hence are unusually vulnerable to disease and injury.
Smallpox, tuberculosis, malaria, and a host of diseases long under control in advanced nations threaten millions of people in developing
nations.

The economic costs of these inadequate systems of health care have
been clearly identified. In the United States, for example, every case
of mental retardation prevented saves some three quarters of a million
dollars in costs of lifetime care and lost income. Every dollar spent on
rehabilitation returns between $17 and $35 to the economy. In Europe
it is estimated that disabilities reduce the economically active population
by about 35% to 28%, a costly portion of so large a work force.
The Soviet Union reports that for every ruble spent during an
11-year national poliomyelitis-vaccination campaign, 67 rubles were
saved for the national economy.

Disease, injuries, and pestilence can be counted in economic terms
in the cost of treatment per patient, the cost of long-term maintenance
and public welfare payments, the loss of projected income and tax
income, and so on. That hundreds of millions of people suffer malnutrition, lack of sanitary environments, and the simplest protection
against disease is a measure of the enormous economic cost and the
task confronting all nations.

Less than 2% of any developing nation's health and medical funds
come from aid programs originating outside the country. Most developed nations have failed to initiate aid programs which expend up
to 0.7% of their gross national product (GNP), as recommended by
the United Nations. Official aid programs from the developed to the
developing countries declined from 0.54% of their GNPs in 1961 to
approximately 0.39% at the end of the decade. During the same period,
domestic savings accounted for 85% of the total investment in developing countries—considerably more than had been required during

the 19th century when the United States and other countries were undergoing their initial development. These trends have continued into the 1970s and in some cases have accelerated.

Realistically, capital for the bulk of developmental purposes, including expanded health care, will have to come from the developing countries themselves—from funds generated by the developmental projects implemented by these countries. In most of these nations health-care needs must compete with more materialistic demands, often in highly political situations. The problem is complicated by the skepticism of many who doubt the contributions that health measures can make to economic development. Health and education have had a relatively low priority in developing nations. Transportation, communications, power, and industry offer more dramatic, visible, and easily measured results in conventional economic terms.

Many surveys by the WHO have detailed the areas of high priority medical care of developing countries:

1) Prevention and control of disease
2) Personal health-care services for rural areas, the deprived, and other segments of the population
3) Maternal and child-health care
4) Education and training of medical and allied personnel
5) Environmental health services

It will be difficult for most of these countries to accomplish all this without assistance in various forms from the developed nations. However limited, national and multilateral direct aid will continue, but the role of foreign private investment is growing and can increase its contribution by erecting the basic economic structure required to support not only health but educational and other social programs as well.

HEALTH AND ECONOMICS

Efforts to extend the benefits of modern medicine globally and nongovernmental participation in worldwide development are major components of a truly historic development—the growing interdependence of all nations. It is not merely a matter of growing global economic interdependence, but interdependence in communications, technology, agriculture, the arts, finance, education, and, of course, medicine. Isolation in any sphere is no longer possible; it is dangerous to pursue it.

Although medicine and economics may appear initially to have little in common, important links bind them closely. Without a healthy work force productivity suffers. Without growing productivity, the resources to sustain or expand medical care fall short of the need. In a world in which human resources are abundant while other resources grow scarce it is not only economically wasteful, it is immoral to ignore health needs.

In economic terms good health services tend to stabilize population growth and contribute to increased productivity. Strong preventive care tends to isolate, if not eradicate, epidemic diseases, thus sustaining employment and growth and avoiding the huge direct and indirect costs of widespread epidemics. Nationwide systems of health delivery tend to stabilize populations under national governments, and economic advancement requires political stability. Good health care creates a more confident, alert work force. Just as health cannot be isolated from other socioeconomic factors in the developmental process, so industry, agriculture, education, and so on cannot be isolated from the health component.

Since private foreign investment is playing an increasingly larger economic role in development—an indirect but important contributory role in building adequate systems of health-care—there must be a recognition of the vital human element in the scheme of development.

Most corporations today accept the principle that human resources constitute their most vital asset. Apart from humanitarian values, there are practical reasons for this viewpoint. For example, there are small differences in products made by different manufacturers. The real differences are in how products and services are distributed; that essentially involves the human element.

Consequently, much time is spent finding and developing the people to run international enterprises. More than half of Citicorp's employees are foreign nationals working in some 98 countries. The company pursues the same personnel-management practices wherever it operates. We must be concerned with all the factors necessary to attract and retain people who are the products of many cultures. Above all, we must follow enlightened practices in the field of human relations.

Theories and practical approaches to this end abound. One of the more widely accepted was put forth by Douglas MacGregor, author of *The Human Side of Enterprise*, a classic work in the management of human resources. MacGregor outlined an ascending order of individual human needs to which he urged corporations to attend in managing their employees. MacGregor describes six categories of physiological and psychological needs which all humans, knowingly or unknowingly, strive to achieve. Each level must be largely mastered before ascending to the next.

The first level of needs which he describes are the basic physiological ones for water, food, rest, and so on. The second level consists of the safety needs for protection from outright danger or the threat of deprivation. Persons living at these lower levels obviously have little time for anything but survival. They cannot be expected to engage in political processes, train for a productive role in modern economy, or practice long-range health maintenance. Too many people in too many places are still trapped at these levels today. The primary thrust of development must be to lift them to higher levels.

MacGregor's third level consists of the social needs: the desire to belong and for association with one's peers. Next comes the need for self-esteem (the fourth level), and then for status, or for appreciation and recognition by others (the fifth level).

Finally, at the sixth and highest level, comes the need for self-fulfillment, an intensely personal realization of one's own potential. A person achieving this state of maximum self-expression is at his most productive. One must surmise that few people attain this state in an absolute way.

MacGregor constructed his analysis to refute the so-called "theory of economic man," the carrot-and-stick approach to managing people. According to this idea, widely accepted in the western world for decades—and still too prevalent I fear—man shuns work. He must be enticed to it by economic reward, driven to it by threat, or both.

In the context of MacGregor's hierarchy of needs one can understand why most institutions, public or private, have elaborate benefit programs covering employees' retirement, education, health, and other requirements. They are part of an effort to help the employee climb the hierarchial ladder of needs.

An examination of the demands of labor in the light of these needs can be revealing. While negotiations or strikes may be publicly depicted as differences over wages, a closer look may cast them in a different light. For example, the perennial battle of policemen and firemen with city governments over which group deserves to earn more because of respective occupational hazards is really not over money but over what MacGregor would call needs of status or self-esteem. The same observation has become increasingly true of other labor negotiations, although I hasten to add that in today's inflationary times money is often the principal issue. In short, monetary issues are often relatively easily settled; difficulties arise over issues that go beyond basic remuneration and job security.

MacGregor's analysis, or any similar later theory, is more difficult to follow in practice than the old theory of economic man. Interpersonal relations of supervisor and employee are critical. Simply applying modern behavioral techniques in the spirit of the theory of economic man will fail, since the techniques appear to employees simply as manipulation. To achieve maximum results, there must be a genuine understanding and appreciation of human behavior and needs.

Health care is a vital component in the process; this is obvious at the lower levels of human needs and no less important at the higher levels. A nation's developmental planning, involving its important human-resource component, must also take these needs into account. By doing so the relation of health and development come clearly into focus.

Populations struggling for their next meal, threatened by disease and plagues which were conquered by stronger nations long ago, and burdened by physical weakness and mental ignorance cannot possibly lift themselves from the drudgery of mere survival to nationbuilding. Good health and reliable, broadly based health-care maintenance are crucial to the establishment of positive mental attitudes among populations pursing the developmental imperative.

Toward a Global Economy

Health, education, and all the other elements of our socioeconomic lives are inextricably interwoven with the developing global economy which Peter Drucker has called the one great achievement of the post-World War II years. Governments and a growing list of international business firms were the first to recognize this blunt reality, but it is now fast intruding upon the lives of people everywhere. For this reason, all health programs—whether in the United States, Japan, Italy, Ghana, Burma, or Bolivia—must be viewed in their global context. The day is past when nations could pursue strictly national economic interests. Self-sufficiency in human and natural resources is beyond the capability of a single nation. The entire global community strains to meet the exigencies of a world of infinite demands and finite resources.

The Bretton Woods Agreement which was adopted after World War II stimulated international commerce that now increases annually at twice the rate of the GNP of the major trading nations. United States international trade has climbed to more than 10% of our GNP in recent years, a point at which any substantial disruption in the flow would create serious problems of unemployment, declining income, and production. The United States is becoming as dependent on international commerce as other advanced countries have been historically.

Only 41 years ago a president of the United States said that tariffs were "solely a domestic question," inappropriate for international bargaining. Today no advanced country dares to adjust tariffs without first consulting its trading partners, and in many instances these matters have been fixed through international agreement in such vehicles as the General Agreement on Tariffs and Trade. Not only tariffs, but import and export licenses, quotas and subsidies, the level of foreign-exchange rates, the price and quality of air and sea transportation, the price of commodities and minerals, fishing rights, and use of the seas are covered by international commitments. Foreign aid is shifting largely to a multilateral basis through the World Bank and various international regional banking institutions. International technical assistance is pooled through agencies of the United Nations.

The International Monetary Fund and the Organization for Economic Cooperation and Development have generated well-entrenched habits of international consultation and persuasion on such domestic subjects as internal interest rates, monetary and fiscal policy, and employment and income policy. Within the European Economic Community and other regional groups the discussions probe more deeply still. Clearly, once jealously guarded national prerogatives are being given over to international debate—willingly or unwillingly.

The reason for this is that international interdependency is increasing at an ever-accelerating pace. It has been brought home to us most dramatically with our sudden plunge into the energy crisis. Oil reserves are unevenly distributed throughout the world, with more than half of known reserves located under the desert sands of the Middle East. Over the next six years imports of this essential resource by the United States will increase from approximately 35% currently to approximately 50 to 60%.

Oil is only the first of many shortages of resources to come. In the last 23 years we have consumed more raw materials than has been used by man prior to 1950, and by 2000 A.D. the demand for almost every mineral will be more than three to five times what it is today. The president's Materials Policy Commission estimated that by 2000 A.D. we shall have to import minerals totaling about $100 billion in 1971 dollars —slightly more than our total trade last year—only half of which will be in oil.

The scarcity of food is another mounting problem. The benefits of the green revolution have already been largely accounted for. As world-wide income continues to rise so too does the quality and quantity of food consumed. Grain is the principal food of the world. Worldwide consumption of grain averages only 400 pounds per capita yearly, while in the United States it averages about one ton. The consumption of grain will soar, not only from increased direct consumption, but also from the expanded production of meat—the increased consumption of which is closely related to improvements in income. Merely to keep pace with population growth for the next generation, to keep feeding populations at their current level will require a doubling of food production.

Minerals and food are the most immediate and dramatic examples of the many problems that require international solutions on a scale the world has never witnessed before. Allocation of resources, planning, production, marketing, finance, training, education and, of course, health all must assume global dimensions if progress is to be maintained.

To deal with these almost colossal problems we must first resolve the difficulties which inevitably surround the institutions and methods whereby global solutions are undertaken. The Bretton Woods Agreement ably served a world in which the dollar was without peer. Today the recovery of the war-devasted economies of the industrial nations, coupled with the emergence of scores of new nations, requires new, more fundamental solutions.

The process is well advanced. Negotiations have been under way for several years, centered largely around the International Monetary Fund, to seek more permanent solutions to the problems plaguing the international monetary system. Substantial progress has been made in developing policies and mechanisms to bring the volatile fluctuations of international currencies under control. Much is left to be done amid a growing awareness that once carefully guarded national economic prerogatives are now legitimate subjects for international debate and regulation.

We are witnessing the inevitable extension of man's efforts to work communally, first through the formation of the city-state, then the nation-state, into the first primitive stages of regionalism, followed closely by the rising pressures of global interdependence.

Ashton, describing the objectives of the industrial revolution in 19th century England, stated the case in the narrow focus of that time: "The central problem of the age was how to feed and clothe and employ generations outnumbering by far those of any earlier time." He described the transformation of basic economic factors in England from individual craftsmen into large-scale production for national markets wherein the workers were anonymous.

A similar transition was going on in the United States. "Localism was yielding ground before the invasion of new laws, customs, institutions and social problems national in scope," wrote Charles and Mary Beard. "The trend of thought and interest was toward a more consolidated national union and a fuller realization of the opportunities for the life commodious and abundant on this continent," they observed.

Peter Drucker described the United States of the late 19th century even more plainly. "The individual acted as a producer and consumer within a continental American market rather than as a 'cosmopolitan' New Yorker or Virginian."

Today we would no more think of raising barriers to interstate commerce than we would of dismantling our productive capacities brick by brick. Yet some people would quickly do this to international trade and other aspects of global interdependence.

What the Beards and Drucker saw occurring in the United States in the 19th century can be extended easily to a global dimension today. We must develop new means to secure our economic future; to do this we must extend our view beyond national boundaries. The recognition of the global interdependence of all people has become essential to our survival.

FOREIGN INVESTMENT AND THE GLOBAL PROSPECT

Within the global view, the contribution of foreign private investment will play a crucial role in the economic advancement of developing countries. How well foreign investment and developing nations work together will bear directly on the success of efforts to improve health and to deal with other critical shortages in the socioeconomic life of much of the world's inhabitants.

For those directly engaged in extending health services to developing countries I shall describe the role of the multinational corporation in a global economy as viewed by a member of one of its oldest and most committed international financial institutions.

The multinational or transnational corporation is a principal result of the process of globalization. Its ranks grow steadily and its members have national origins as diverse among the advanced nations as the products and services which these corporations dispense. Not by design, but simply as a result of the process of globalization itself, the multinational corporation has been cast in the forefront of this incredibly rapid development. As with all bearers of change, the multinational firm is often charged with being the cause of the frustrations and fears that rapid change inevitably induces in the souls of many.

The growth of the multinational corporation was inevitable. Transatlantic crossings were reduced from four days to seven hours in the two decades following World War II. International trade volume increased threefold between 1953 and 1965. Daily consultations between governments, financiers, marketeers, engineers, and assorted business strategists on different continents have become commonplace. Integrated computers on different continents work simultaneously at the same problems. A drop in the exchange rate of the dollar in London is instant news in New York and Tokyo. Accumulated information on markets within individual countries flows voluminously between continents. International travel is no longer an upper-class luxury but a middle-class necessity. International tourism is a new and major world industry. Quantum gains in technology have opened broad new channels for the global exchange of ideas.

All of this has forced a wholesale breakdown in barriers to trade, payments, and capital flow between countries and an explosion in the international exchange of goods, services, money, people, and ideas. The principal vehicle for this flow is the multinational corporation. It alone possessses the large-scale organization, skills, and experiences to expedite such a massive transfer of goods, commerce, technology, and ideas.

Since the multinational corporation is most easily identifiable among the swirl of change wrought by the globalization process, it is most often resented and vilified by those who cannot observe the entire process and tend to deal with the world in Manichaean simplicities. What we see are manifestations of the forces that prompted national industries and a continental market in the United States in the last century now working to extend industries and markets to the entire world. This is happening to all nations. The technological possibilities of the day make global strategies essential if we are to achieve the economies of scale necessary to employ scarce resources most efficiently. More urgently, it is essential to our long-term survival. Developing the raw materials still available to us alone will require enormous amounts of capital. Single projects of half a billion dollars and more are beyond the capacity of one multinational organization. Such projects increasingly will require broad international participation.

Global economic interdependence manifests itself in countless subtle ways. A simple example will prove this. Copper mined in western Africa is shipped to Germany, where it is used to make electrical wiring installed in elevators manufactured in Belgium and sold to a British construction firm building a hotel for a United States joint venture with a Latin American country. Construction materials come from local sources and a neighboring country. Linen, some dinnerware, and furniture from Hong Kong, Japan, and Taiwan, respectively—where Indonesian hardwoods are used—decorate the hotel. The architect is Brazilian, some earth-moving equipment used in construction was made in Illinois, and so on. Tourists and businessmen from all over the world make up most of the guests.

To bring it home more directly, United States farm exports are a case in point. Last year these soared to more than $13 billion—grain from the Midwest, soybeans from the Southeast, cotton from the Southwest, etc.—and the prospects in light of growing world demand are staggering. Tracing the impact of this trade into tertiary industries, we see a host of neighoring services and businesses in farm communities benefiting. Stability and expansion of global commerce are of growing importance to orderly economic development in every corner of our nation.

The steps taken in one nation will have immediate effects in other countries, and these effects will multiply. When the rediscount rate rises in New York the cost of money may rise in Brussels. Price controls in the United States send American fertilizer production into export markets. A strike at a Volkswagen plant in Germany increases sales in the United States of both American and Japanese small cars.

We need more sophisticated global intelligence systems to provide early warnings of possible emergencies. If crises continue to creep up on us, we may soon find ourselves overwhelmed. New intelligence systems must account for the discrepancies between political and economic realities.

Raymond Vernon has said, "There is a stubborn life and purpose in the system of nation-states, and there is a tenacious capacity on the part of mankind to disregard the seemingly inevitable." He worries that we may be in another of those "period[s] of revulsion from the international order before the world is prepared to move on to a new international synthesis." If so, we must avoid lingering too long in such a period. We have a problem with only one solution: to accept, encourage, and work within a global framework. If we fail to make this basic commitment, to debate and compromise our various positions within it, then we doom ourselves to a new dark age.

FOREIGN INVESTMENT AND DEVELOPING COUNTRIES

It obviously follows that international programs of health care are essential on a global scale. Health care is integrally bound to the economic prospects of developing countries and to the role that foreign private investment can play in their development. How private foreign corporations relate to developing countries, using my corporation's experience as an example, may prove helpful to those working to expand health-care services within these countries.

Seventy-two years of operating abroad has taught us one lesson well: Whatever a foreign corporation does in the way of business must benefit the host country. If it does not, the corporation will fail in its business objectives. It must interpret its business in terms of what the host country expects of foreign capital. Quite often that is spelled out in official development planning.

By examining such plans and talking with government officials the corporation can determine where its activities lend support. Corporations are not charitable organizations; what they do earns a profit. But corporations must also accomplish the host's objectives better than any other system. If they do not do so, private investment will not survive in any country for long.

My corporation engages in some activities that are marginally profitable but are of sound public purpose. We even do some things one might call strictly charitable. But we are not organized to sustain these activities, and it would be a delusion to think that our activities will contribute importantly to changing the world or even will make a substantial difference in the long term. The true measure of our work anywhere is how well our profit-making activities work for the public good.

Corporations must carefully examine their relations with host countries. During the debate last year over the role of multinational corporations in Chile my institution examined what its role had been there and, in a larger perspective, what our role in other countries is and should be. As a result, four basic, simple principles were communicated to our worldwide branches:

1) We must never lose sight of the fact that we are guests in foreign countries. We must conduct ourselves accordingly. We recognize the right of governments to pass legislation and our obligation to conform.

2) Under these circumstances, we recognize that we can survive only if we successfully demonstrate to local authorities that our presence is beneficial.

3) Every country must find its own way politically and economically. Whether we believe that local policies are wise or not, we should try to function as best we can under prevailing conditions.

4) We feel free to discuss matters directly affecting our interests with local governments, but we recognize that they have final regulatory authority.

We have no rules carved in stone, but these four are all but etched in granite on the board-room floor.

Banks do get involved in developmental planning as consultants on international finance and as providers of capital. With the declining role of foreign aid worldwide, the private sector of the economy has borne an increasing share of funding developmental projects in basic industry and infrastructure. The governments of developing nations have become major clients, and negotiations with clients in manufacturing and service industries usually involve discussions with public officials of the recipient host country.

Health programs and projects are well known to my bank; we have helped with their financing in many countries. We have negotiated the financing of hospitals and hospital equipment in many nations. In some countries we operate family installment-loan programs at modest interest rates to assist in the delivery of dental and general medical services to low-income groups. We conduct similar programs elsewhere aimed at making prescription drugs available to those of modest income. Our overseas offices regularly participate in blood-donation and similar drives. In cooperation with local authorities, we have inaugurated drug-control campaigns in several countries where drug abuse has become a problem. We have helped finance sewage and sanitation improvements and sometimes we have donated pumping or water-treatment equipment on a small scale to neighborhoods where the only water which had been available was contaminated.

Because everywhere we are among the more heavily regulated components of the private sector of the economy, banks maintain close, almost daily, communications with host governments. Consequently, our officers must be part diplomat, part banker. We are more involved with government than most businessmen working abroad. The same parallel has been drawn between medicine and diplomacy. It is a characteristic of global interdependency that relations among countries increasingly touch the lives of many citizens. This new participatory diplomacy may never replace the historic, formal lines of communications, but it may well come to equal them in impact.

A final word about our operations in developing countries. We are entering a period in which the second generation of leaders after independence are taking control of governments. This generation is usually well-educated and sophisticated in modern finance, government, and the ways of the world. The heady nationalism quite naturally generated during the years of struggle for independence is of secondary importance to this new breed.

More pragmatic, if less charismatic, than their predecessors, the new leaders are less wedded to ideology than to the practical pursuit of building a nation. They offer great hope, far more than has been generally noted amid the prevailing despair about inflation, shortages of resources, and other global problems. People, after all, constitute our most valuable resource in the struggle for a better world, and its adaptability to change is well known. I have great confidence in the leaders of the developing countries.

William Faulkner expressed it more than two decades ago when, in accepting the Nobel Prize for literature, he said, "Man will not endure, he will prevail." This must become a global credo.

WORLD HEALTH AND WORLD HUNGER:
PUTTING DEVELOPMENT ETHICS
TO THE TEST

DENIS GOULET, PH.D. (POL. SCI.)

Visiting Fellow, Overseas Development Council

T HE vicious circle of poverty is a familiar image. In its many variations the theme is that people are poor because they are not productive, they are not productive because they are not well-fed, they are not well-fed because they are not productive, and they are not productive because they are poor. There exists another kind of circle, however, which is little mentioned and no less distressing: the "closed circle" of our thinking about development. If we are to judge from salient themes in recent discussions of development —resource shortages and food aid to starving masses—we may have come full circle to views voiced thirty years ago when international officials, financiers and experts first started talking about development.

The notion then prevailing was that rich nations could help war damaged, and later poor, nations industrialize by transferring investment capital, food, and other supplies to them. Because it stressed assistance, this outlook came to be termed the *assistentialist* approach.

As time passed, it grew obvious that this view of reality was too simplistic. A more basic *developmental* approach replaced it, stressing the need to modernize structures and infra-structures of production and decision-making. Development was portrayed as a series of stages through which poor societies, with help from outside, could lift themselves up or, to use Walt Rostow's phrase, "take off" into self-sustained growth. But this image too fell victim to time and to a more critical spirit.

Scholars alert to the dependency systems used by the rich to keep subservient the underdeveloped poor brought a new term into development's linguist arena. It was *liberation*: economic improvement of the entire population through radical change aimed at abolishing the dependency of national societies on outside forces and the subordination of their popular masses to native elites allied to those forces.

Three successive terminologies have thus dominated the development debate: assistentialism, developmentalism and liberation. Each new emphasis criticized omissions or distortions of the prior one without, however, necessarily rejecting all components of the former language. Developmentalists, although preaching the need for new economic and administrative structures, did not deny the need for relief in times of calamity—drought, floods, volcanic eruptions. Similarly, liberation theorists, while centering on political struggle to alter power relations, did not reject the developmental goal of increasing production and efficiency.

As Americans now focus their attention on resource shortages, world hunger and health, they must not let themselves be lulled into a new kind of "assistentialist" thinking about development. So many discussions of development and of U.S./Third World relations are preempted by themes of food, fuel and fertilizer that the danger arises of seeing world development simply as a matter of food aid to starving nations or of compensatory financial assistance to offset inflationary price rises.

This is why I have spoken of a "closed circle": post World War II assistentialism, developmentalism, liberation, and now a new version of assistentialism which can easily mystify the issues. But hunger and ill health are merely dramatic symptoms of a deeper ill: the persistence of national and international orders which foster distorted development. Consequently, the problem is not met solely by boosting food aid or by cutting births but, ultimately, by creating new ground rules governing access to the world's productive resources. Societies now powerless must gain such access *upstream*—at the production end—and not merely *downstream*—at the distribution end—if an equitable, dynamic, and liberating form of world development is to appear. But a new social compact for humanity cannot be created in a vacuum; initial steps must be taken by solving concrete problems such as starvation, inadequate health care, and resource shortages. What is crucial is the *mode* of solution adopted. Otherwise stated, the present international order must be altered if we are to avoid mere palliatives.

These general remarks on development serve as background for raising three questions which determine one's view of world hunger and health. These questions are:

—what is the basis for human solidarity?

—which social forces control the transition to a new world order and what values do they promote? and

—how can limited problem-solving to meet world hunger and promote health avoid being palliative and deal with causes?

THE BASIS OF WORLDWIDE SOLIDARITY

Solidarity is the primary ethical value one must appeal to in dealing with these problems. It is a more fundamental moral category than either justice or charity. Solidarity is a major developmental value to be promoted within rich, food-laden countries if they are not to be anti-developed. Similarly, it is a central value to be concretized in needy areas if some measure of justice is to be achieved. In view of its central importance, I wish to examine in detail the foundations of universal human solidarity as ethical value.

Modern communications render isolation among human societies impossible. More than forty years ago Lewis Mumford wrote that "the joint stock of knowledge and technical skill transcends the boundaries of individual or national egos, and to forget that fact is not merely to enthrone superstition but to undermine the essential planetary basis of technology itself."[1] And French economist François Perroux adds that "technical conditions for the establishment of a planetary economy now exist."[2] No country can erect walls around itself without thereby destroying the international foundations of technology. Technological production and the resulting consumption of its goods are rapidly unifying the globe. Human dreams are everywhere affected by the standardizing promise of technology; and the homogenization of behavior is well under way, especially among the world's businessmen, professionals, technicians, and bureaucrats.

More significant than converging behavioral patterns, however, are the general images gaining ascendancy in the world: technology projects visions of material betterment, control over nature, and of society's ability to affect the direction and speed of its change processes. Beyond technology's unifying effect lie three deeper foundations of human solidarity.

a) Human beings are one by their common humanity. Although thinkers differ over the meaning of "human," each makes universal claims. All agree that beyond differences of race, nationality, culture, or social organization a common "humanness" is present. Their common humanity is, therefore, the first ontological basis for solidarity among all men and women.

b) A second foundation is the common occupation of the planet by all human organisms. Throughout its physical extension, the earth is governed by identical laws and is subject to the same indeterminisms. Despite variations in climate, relief and geography, this planet has a specific identity distinct from other cosmic bodies. All humanity dwells on one planet. The symbiosis between human beings and "nature" presupposes an intimate link between the two. Each person is part of nature and the world of objects. Were it otherwise, they could not be treated as mere "objects" by others. Moreover, physical occupation of this planet is the lot of all persons, not only of some. Even if human beings do not interact directly with their fellow human beings, they are related at least *indirectly*, thanks to their common links to the same planetary system. The prospects opened up by recent space exploration in no way modify the organic relations tying every human being to this planet as to their cosmic home so long as they are born on this earth and dwell here. Were permanent emigration to other planets to take place in the future, human solidarity would acquire an expanded basis—namely, the unity of cosmic planetary systems instead of a single planet. In either case, human beings are interdependent because of identical ties to one system, planetary or cosmic.

c) Along with their common humanity and their ties to one cosmic environment, a third basis of solidarity exists among humans: their unity of destiny. Whatever be their personal occupations—farmers, students, news reporters, politicians, artists, machinists, persons who tend the home, or salespersons—all must fulfill themselves in a human mode. All philosophical systems postulate, at least implicitly, a common destiny for humanity: the fate of one is the fate of all. The universality of human destiny represents no sectarian point of view, but the common patrimony of human thought.

Nevertheless, human beings rarely translate their existential solidarity into cooperative behavior: they consistently act *as though they were not bound together in webs of solidarity*. Partisan claims assert themselves as though they had general merit. Classes, nations, and individuals seek to dominate other classes, nations, and individuals. And although lip service is given to the "common good of humanity" or to world community, development problems continue to be defined through the prisms of parochial mercantile, strategic, or ideological interests. Even within international organizations, solidarity is often sacrificed to narrow political interests. Men and women have not yet learned how to respond to the exigencies of solidarity written into their very being.

Paradoxically, genuine solidarity can be won only after much conflict. One source of conflict is the uneven development found in the world. Nations once colonized or still economically dominated need to assert their nationalism virulently in order to do battle against underdevelopment. Highly industrialized nations, on the other hand, need to limit their own exercise of sovereignty if harmful domination effects are to be neutralized. Identical norms cannot be applied to all countries. To illustrate, non-industrial countries need high tariffs to nurture fragile incipient industry, whereas industrialized countries must lower tariffs to admit Third World goods to buyers' markets. Equity requires that compensatory standards be followed so as to assure meeting priority needs. Unless all countries endorse solidarity, however, these standards will appear irrational, unjust, or threatening to some. Consequently, the manner in which we view conflict assumes decisive importance.

Conservatives generally presume social harmony to be normal, and conflict to be subversive. Their underlying assumption is that existing institutions are just or, at least, that they are the lesser evil among all realistic alternatives. Reality in most underdeveloped lands contradicts this view, however. Here basic structures are often unjust and devoid of legitimacy, despite a facade of legality. Social conflict thus becomes necessary to challenge established disorder. And because solidarity implies powers of self-disposition in those who practice it, disharmony becomes a prelude to development.

The dynamism of conflict brings to the surface an even deeper tension which exists between the demands of justice and those of peace.

The dilemma is this: peace comes to mean stabilizing the present world order, largely through collegiate decisions of the big powers. But this order is structurally unjust, for as Myrdal tells us, the theory of international trade had as its purpose the *"explaining away of the international equality problem."*[3] Therefore, those aiming at creating just structures, in many nations as in the world at large, must do battle against the present social order. Inasmuch as the stewards of this order are also the world's peace managers, however, those dedicated to social justice sometimes endanger peace. Even they recognize, however, that certain kinds of violence might annihilate the human species or destroy the minimum institutional fabric from which a new world order might be constructed once the old order were destroyed.

Although development is a two-edged sword, both a good thing and a dangerous thing, human beings cannot abdicate their historic task: to build a world of authentic development for all.

Present power distribution in the world system favors societies already endowed with disproportionate wealth and influence. This is why Third World leaders increasingly repudiate solidarity with a world system which victimizes them and brings more advantages to the donors of "aid" than to the recipients. Accordingly, the planned use of vital resources is the only rational approach to world development. The late Bengali mystic and poet, Tagore, believed that only what is compatible with the universal has permanent survival value; anything less is doomed to perish.[4] He may be right, since even technological research cannot keep pace with expanding acquisitive instincts. Once development's benefits are universally desired, the appropriation of goods on any basis other than universal human solidarity in the face of needs is not a viable ethic.

Neither individualism nor collectivism, if taken absolutely or in isolation from other values, can provide sound principles of development. The first renders justice impossible, the second integral human maturation. Some optimal blend of entrepreneurship, allied to projective identification with group interests by social creators, is required if social change is to generate increased solidarity, both within nations and in the world at large.

As applied to inequities in food use and health care, the principle of solidarity decrees the elimination of waste and luxury among the rich, so as to meet the urgent needs of the poor. The late Brazilian geographer Josué de Castro, author of *Geography of Hunger*, when reflecting twenty years ago on the five-to-one ratio of cereal grains consumed in producing meat for human consumption, remarked that "to eat meat is to practice cannibalism: it is to devour our fellow humans."

We need something far more drastic than a shift in lifestyles or consumption patterns among citizens of developed nations. Our global economic and political institutions must be revamped to allocate resources on the basis of priority needs. The present international economic order operates from an opposite principle, that of the market place: goods go to those with effective purchasing power. Most rem-

edies proposed to correct economic inequities tackle the problem
downstream, at the distribution end. What is necessary, on the contrary,
is to challenge the rules of access to resources *upstream*, at the production end. Recent schemes to recirculate oil dollars or offer compensatory financing to offset inflation simply ignore this issue. Accordingly,
such measures, taken as a whole, constitute a strategy of domestication
of the Third World. No effort is made to create new ethical rules for
access to resources in the light of planetary solidarity. Instead we are
offered philanthropic transfers aimed at forestalling revolutionary up-
risings destructive of the privileges of the opulent. Yet solidarity cannot
be genuine or long-lasting unless it is founded on reciprocal strength in
bargaining positions. The present international system is not some sac-
rosanct, fragile vessel enabling us to navigate perilous waters. On the
contrary, it is the creation of an obsolete elite designed by them before
the world's oppressed peoples had launched their historic cry—"No
more domination, no more domestication!" The international order
must not be protected; it must be radically transformed.

The Stewards of the Transition

But who will preside over the transformation? Who will be the stewards of the transition? This is no idle question: spokesmen for the great
powers, for multinational corporations and for other international elite
groups constantly appeal to solidarity among nations to solve global
problems. One need not object to their metaphors—global village or
world community. But one is entitled to question whether their kind of
solidarity can lead to reciprocity and equity among nations. Or does
their conception of the "global village" require that they retain their
privileged status as "village elders"?

Within this context, it is illuminating to compare diverse scenarios
for the transition to a new world order. In the words of Richard Falk,
an international law scholar from Princeton University:

> We are in the midst of a world order transition from the state
> system to some form of central guidance. In my view, the most
> probable outcome of transition, as matters now stand, is likely
> to be a world order pattern that is even more dangerous, ex-
> ploitative, and repressive than the state system.

A grim prospect! Yet Falk insists that:

such an undesirable outcome, although the most probable
course of events, is not yet by any means inevitable.[5]

Many futurists uncritically endorse an image of politics as the art of
the possible, interpreting this art as the skillful manipulation of present
and future possibilities, within existing or predictable boundaries. Yet
development politics is the art of creating new possibilities, of shatter-
ing existing parameters and opening the way for new ones. This is the
lesson we have learned from Mao, from Nyerere, from Velasco. Attempts to create new social possibilities can, it is true, be crushed by
counter forces, witness Chile, September 1973. And both our former
Ambassador to the U.N., John Scali, and our present Ambassador,
Daniel Moynihan, have threatened Third World nations with un-
specified sanctions if they try to rewrite international debating rules too
drastically. In stark terms, the ethical issues at play are reducible to
two: which social forces will be the stewards of the emerging world
order? and on what values will the new international order be built?

For John Scali, Henry Kissinger, multinational managers, and most
international relations scholars, it is self-evident that the transition process ought to be managed by "responsible, non-revolutionary" elites
like themselves.

But for President Boumedienne of Algeria, OPEC leaders, and other
actors in the world arena, it is equally clear that the architects of the
new order should include leaders of revolutionary governments and
movements, non-governmental organizations with a popular base, and
other pressure groups committed to social justice. They hope to
counter the greater influence of today's world elite by adding to their
coalition the forces represented by populists in key industrialized countries, dissident bureaucrats, technicians, professionals, and military
men. Those whom Falk calls the "global populists," however, cannot
influence the evolution of the international order except through the
mediation of such organized groups as OPEC, the Group of 77 at
UNCTAD, and Third World voting blocks in the U.N.

Of more importance than the actors, however, are their values, and
the prospects for subordinating their interests to the requirements of
global justice, peace, ecological integrity, and equitable power distribution.

Underlying all efforts to create a world order in which world hunger
can be abolished and world health improved is the need to limit con-

sumption. Erich Fromm judges the alienation of affluence to be no less dehumanizing than alienation in misery.[6] Moreover, hunger among starving masses can be permanently abolished only if the privileged rich minority of the human race gives up its present standards of wasteful abundance and restructures its own economic incentives around priority needs. No amount of "trickle down" of its surplus can ever suffice to feed the hungry or enable them to reach a decent level of development.

Austerity or "sufficiency for all" is the watchword for the world at large. The world's hungry masses would welcome this kind of austerity for it assures them something they have never had: the possibility of having enough. Such austerity differs from that imposed by most governments, who have usually proven adept only at tightening the belts of those already in distress. Gandhi never tired of repeating that there are enough goods in the world for everyone's needs, but not for everyone's greed. The developed world—and this includes the privileged strata of the population in poor countries—has legitimized its structures of greed by invoking the necessity, and the merits, of the market system. But an international economic order founded on the market system, even if it mitigates inequities by redistributive actions, is inherently unable to solve the hunger, health, and scarcity problems at their roots.

One has only to contrast the performance of China with that of India in abolishing famine and improving health within their respective borders. Adequate production, conservation, and distribution of food and health services were as difficult to achieve in China as they were in India. Yet China's basic value options, and the incentive systems resulting therefrom, have led it to refuse to face the problem in mercantile terms, or by merely combining market mechanisms with corrective state actions. The mobilization of Chinese society set out to meet the needs of all. In addition, systematic warfare is waged against recurring tendencies exhibited by some to use the economy, the political system, or their own educational advantages to resurrect allocation practices which favor their own interests. Not by accident, therefore, are famine and related diseases absent from China while they still prevail in India.

For architects of a strategy against world hunger and preventable disease the lesson is clear. The world's financial, economic, political, and legal orders must rest, institutionally, on the primacy of moral over material incentives. That is to say, the motor force of international exchanges in an era of scarcity must be the overarching incentive of human solidarity, not the market principle.

A qualitative difference between two conceptions of the market is decisive here. For economic liberals, the market is the organizing principle of productive activity, responsive to effective purchasing power as to its prime stimulus. But, as Karl Mannheim observed,[7] the competitive market need not be an organizing principle; it can simply be a regulatory mechanism to minimize waste, inefficiency, and overcentralization. Even a conservative economist like Henry Wallich[8] asserts that the survival and continued profitability of capitalist firms depends, not on continued private or corporate ownership of the means of production, but on maintaining the market and access to markets by individual firms.

If world market competition could be subordinated to an organizing principle drawn from a political consensus about goals, kinds of goods, and proportional allocations, the way would be open for an international economic order compatible with development and equity for all.

The struggle to create such a world order clearly faces overwhelming odds. "Global populists" have no power to compare with the leverage over events wielded by multinational managers, big power leaders, or international financiers. Moreover, the problem is so pressing that they must adopt immediate measures of assistance, notwithstanding their concern for the quality of the future world order; hence their need to reflect critically on the principles underlying their change strategy. Can any change strategy allow one to solve problems today, while shaping tomorrow's world order so as to eliminate the causes of mass hunger and unnecessary illness? Is it possible to go beyond palliatives?

GOING BEYOND PALLIATIVES

Our search is for leverage points where concrete actions can provide non-palliative solutions to issues of world order and the task is to define a strategy of transition from the present system of decision-making to one which is more just. Not only must the primacy of the market system be overturned; so must the hegemony of great powers and multinational corporations.

These institutions have revealed themselves largely impotent in the face of a wide array of problems ranging from ecological catastrophe and linked resource scarcities, to the threat of species-annihilating warfare or radioactive contamination and the stubborn persistence of the train of ills attaching to underdevelopment—exploitation, domination, repression, starvation. Even the complacent now concede that national, or even regional, solutions are not enough: worldwide actions and institutions have become urgently necessary. A growing consensus is forming around two assertions:

—that the present world order must give way to a new one; and

—that the present order is, in fact, evolving under the pressure of events.

But where is this evolution leading us, towards what kind of world order?

There exist several competing models of a new world order, differentiated by judgments as to who ought to be its major architects and what values they ought to promote. It is worth summarizing here the conclusions reached by Richard Falk and his colleagues in the World Order Models Project:

(1) The state system is being superseded by a series of interlocking social, economic, political, technological, and ecological tendencies which are likely to eventuate in some form of dysutopia or negative utopia, i.e., in a very undesirable and dangerous structure of response to the problems posed by the deepening crisis in the state system.

(2) Although this disquieting outcome seems probable as of now, it is not inevitable. There is also a beneficial option, premised upon an affirmation of the wholeness of the planet and the solidarity of the human species, that could bring about a rearrangement of power, wealth, and authority that would be more beneficial than anything the world has heretofore known.

(3) Initially, the global reform movement needed to underlie such a positive outcome has to take principal shape outside of and mainly in opposition to the centers of constituted political and economic power—it will almost certainly have to be populist and anti-governmental in character and origins. Such a movement should be premised upon non-violence to the extent possible.

(4) The principal initial focus of a movement for positive global reform should involve education-for-action, that is, demonstrating that the felt needs and frustrations of people in a variety of concrete social circumstances around the world arise from the inability of governmen-

tal or multinational actors to find short-range, middle-level, and long-range solutions to the distresses and dangers of our world.

(5) The case for global reform should be premised on a basic assessment of structural trends and options. It need not rest altogether on the collison course conveniently being programmed by apocalyptic reformers to take effect by the year 2000.[9]

My intent here is not to review the evidence for this view, but rather to explore how we can best equip ourselves with the conceptual tools we need to reflect, both critically and creatively, on the ethical and global dimensions of world hunger and disease. To do so, we need to understand how small incremental or gradual steps can contribute to creating a new world order. The question is ancient but ever-contemporaneous: can any actions I take be anything other than palliative measures or make a difference? Zen teachers are fond of reminding us that to "lift a finger is to move the universe." When so many others with wealth, power, and influence are moving their arms and their bodies (to say nothing of their computers, capital, and equipment) to create a hierarchical world order serving market interests, we have no excuse for *not* lifting a finger. One responsibility remains with us, nonetheless: to assure that even our incremental steps help create new possibilities.

We must, at the outset, break with prevailing and projected models or paradigms of world order. Accordingly, some of the changes to be pursued will constitute a social mutation.

Moreover, apparently identical measures sometimes constitute mere palliatives whereas, in different circumstances, they creatively expand possibilities for future change. Two opposing kinds of incrementalism can be identified: the one palliative, the other creative.

Palliatives block deep change by lulling people into accepting minor gradual improvements instead of adequate responses to fundamental problems. As time passes, however, palliatives always worsen the condition they mean to cure, either by raising hopes they cannot satisfy or by tinkering with defective social mechanisms, thereby postponing treatment until the disease becomes incurable. Creative incremental measures, on the contrary, are designed to open new possibilities for subsequent radical change even though at the moment of adoption they appear modest. Such measures contain a latent dynamism which propels society past immediate problem-solving and renders new futures possible. Physicist-philosopher John Wilkinson has remarked that the potential energy of a rock that has been sitting on top of a hill for a million years is harmless to anyone. Only when its energy can be made kinetic by some random push can it cause a new situation to arise. Contemplated social measures, like energy, are endowed with a greater or lesser potential for generating major transformation. A good strategist must learn to discern which measures have but a palliative potential, which a creative potential. All latent social energy remains fruitless until it is kineticized. Of course, the total consequences of a given measure cannot always be assessed before the fact. Randomness or serendipity can transform "safe" concessions into explosively revolutionary instruments. Nonetheless, sensitive change agents can appeal to subjective and objective criteria when they attempt to assess the change potential contained in contemplated moves.

Even those revolutionists who abhor violent methods have lost their faith in the capacity of *existing institutions* to produce required changes in piecemeal fashion. If, therefore, they feel compelled to resort to seemingly incremental tactics, they always do so in the hope that today's modest moves will open the door to deeper mutations tomorrow. Consequently, all specific recommendations made by change agents must be evaluated in the light of the long-term intentions of those same agents. An illustration may help. We may suppose that country "A" favors creating an international ocean regime having sole authority over all seabeds and committed to using the oceans' resources exclusively for peaceful development purposes. Let us further assume that country "A" adopts this scheme because it considers an international ocean regime to be a first step in the direction of abolishing national sovereignties and creating world political responsibility. That country's leaders may reach the practical judgment that the cause of international decision-making is advanced if global control over the oceans can be established before sovereign nations acquire uncontested rights over them. In this case, the measure is not merely palliative: subjectively at least, it is perceived as capable of creating new leverage for a more profound institutional change later.

The identical ocean regime, however, may be supported by country "B" for quite opposite reasons. Country "B" may oppose the prospect of international decision-making and fear the eventual demise of national sovereignty. Nevertheless, the country might wish to curb military or commerical exploitation of the ocean floor by powerful nations to the detriment of poorer nations. Relative to a world guidance system to replace nation-states, the final objective, "B's" support of an international ocean regime, must be considered a mere palliative. In both cases incrementalism is clearly at work, but a subjective criterion helps us discern whether the same measure constitutes palliative or creative incrementalism for its respective agents. More importantly, does any *objective* criterion exist for distinguishing incremental steps which are mere patchwork from those which genuinely expand future possibilities.

British scientist Denis Gabor, author of *Inventing the Future,*is convinced that palliative solutions to social problems, however attractive or adequate they appear at the time of adoption, inevitably worsen the ills they seek to cure. According to Gabor, non-palliative measures, when programmed in a computer designed to isolate the consequences of a contemplated course of action, can be shown in simulated exercises which portray hypothetical possible futures, to result in better conditions. The opposite also holds true: palliatives, once played out, make matters visibly worse. If this be so, one can distinguish palliative from creative incremental measures *without appealing to ideological norms.* Such norms remain decisive, of course, for true believers whether the object of their faith is free-enterprise or socialism. For them there exists one unmistakable criterion of discernment which they allege to be "objective," namely, the degree to which the measure envisaged strengthens or weakens the social system they champion. Great wisdom would doubtless be required of programmers if they are to assess all important factors correctly in their computer-programming exercise. Nevertheless, if Gabor is right, it becomes at least theoretically possible to judge the change potential of prospective measures. In fact, one can create a scale on which to measure the potential transformation value of all steps proposed.

A word must be added to explain why palliative solutions to social ills are so pernicious. Solutions of this type do not root out the causes of social ailments but merely tamper with symptoms. Politically speaking, they are designed to "buy off" potential agents of deeper change with social bribes, in the form of visible benefits. Yet, the mode in which development is pursued determines whether societies will be liberated or alienated at the end of the development road. The manner itself is as decisive as the matter, the *how* as the *what.* Many of development's benefits can be obtained in an elitist, technocratic, oligarchic mode even under the ostensible flag of greater freedom and democracy. Behind the scenes, however, may lurk deterministic forces manipulating mass opinion and desires. To achieve the benefits of development while sacrificing human freedom and critical intelligence, is, however, to negate the good life and the good society which development professes to nurture. Palliative measures may solve problems or settle issues, but they cannot foster those qualities in life which constitute the final goals of development itself.

Since anything less than the basic reconversion of the world's institutions is sheer palliative to the evils of world underdevelopment, the crucial task incumbent upon social change agents is to devise bold measures consonant with feasability and creativity. What becomes increasingly clear, moreover, is that the choice of a development strategy any society makes directly affects that society's impact on the international order in gestation. I lack the time to review alternative strategies defended by competing actors in the development arena. But it is worth recalling three primal images of underdevelopment, to each of which corresponds a preferred strategic path.[10]

A first image is of a straggling procession of countries scurrying to "close the gap." Most weaker nations fall behind: they "can't make it" and become, in the denigrating language used by some Western writers, "the soft states." A second image of international development relations is that of a living pyramid: countries, classes and interest groups on top are able to rise higher and higher because they rest on the shoulders of those under them. Since it is a living structure, this pyramid is continually in movement due to the endemic jostling for position. Periodic upheavals and convulsions lead to a reversal of favored position. This pyramidal image is mirrored both in domestic stratification and in global power distribution. A third image, fast gaining adherents in Western countries, negates the basic assumptions of the first two, namely:

—that long-term expansion of production and consumption are both good and possible; and

—that technology has an unlimited capacity to solve problems.
According to this pessimistic third view, the historical march is headed, not for the Promised Land of Development, but toward the bottomless pit of catastrophe—ecological, biological, psychological, and political.

These primal images determine the criteria for choosing development strategies. All center on value judgments about what is a "better" soci-

ety. They differ, of course, as to the role assigned to leaders and experts or to the masses, the scale of priorities in benefits sought, the
social and human price to be paid for any gains realized, the time span
deemed acceptable before major gains are achieved, the mode in which
change will be stimulated. Underlying all strategies, however, is an
initial choice made about overarching incentive systems. As mentioned
above, the prime motor of economic activity will either be some form
of material incentive, responsive to market mechanisms or planned re-
wards, or primary moral incentives stimulating effort around larger
ideological goals: the abolition of misery, equal justice for all, the conquest of autonomy and dignity. Not by accident have the market nations grown pessimistic about the present world conditions, whereas
the Chinese see the disorder as potentially creative. To them the current world scene is characterized by "great but good disorder." Chinese
historian Paul Lin articulates this viewpoint in the following words:

> There are acute struggles unfolding—between the exploiter
> and the exploited classes within capitalist societies, between
> imperialist powers and the victims of their neocolonialism,
> among the imperialist powers (in particular the superpowers)
> themselves, and between the imperialist powers (including
> today's USSR) and the socialist countries. The intense fury of
> these struggles has torn apart the fabric of the old order . . . .
>
> In the Chinese perception, the essence underlying all this
> sound and fury is that the world is moving at a higher
> metabolic rate in the shedding of the old order and the building
> of the new. The dismantling of old structures always creates
> some disorder, but it is 'disorderly' for the old forces that are
> now gradually receding from their all-powerful roles of the
> world stage, in favour of the newly independent resurgent
> forces of the developing nations. The trend is unfettering and
> moving ahead in the stream of history, and it is in this sense
> that it is good disorder.[11]

Conclusion

As I conclude, some readers may register suprise at my failure to
mention several of the terms currently afloat in the ethical debate particularly over hunger: triage, lifeboat ethics, distributive norms in an
age of scarcity, the role of population control in food policy. Let me

state unequivocally that I regard all these topics as important. Nevertheless, they do not go to the heart of the issue. Here I wish to recall the title of this paper: "World Hunger and World Health: Putting Development Ethics to the Test." Indeed the coexistence of mass starvation and preventable disease alongside wasteful abundance, is the scandalous reality that does go to the heart of the matter. Are we to diagnose mass hunger and ill health as accidents, aberrations, temporary distortions in an otherwise sound system? Or are they but a symptom, a surface manifestation, of the world's structural inequities which render abiding human misery possible even as massive resources are spent to achieve something called "development." Is there anything genuine about this kind of "development"? Or does it not rather constitute some pernicious form of "anti-development"?

Present circumstances do not allow us the luxury of ignoring world hunger and health problems; they place development ethics to the test in several ways.

First, they unmask the quality of our ethics. Is our ethics pious rhetoric or effective *praxis?* Is it a set of conceptual standards for judging ends and evaluating means, or a critical tool in our struggle to translate specific development value options into action?

Second, does our ethical response to starvation and unnecessary illness produce solutions based on human solidarity, seen as a vital ingredient of our own human development? I have in this paper stressed the need to found our response to mass starvation, not primarily on the ethical categories of justice or charity, but on solidarity. Why do I believe the basic category to be solidarity? Because to deny, by our action or inaction, the reality of human solidarity in a time of interdependent scarcity, is to pass ethical judgment on the unworthiness of our own concepts of development.

I have also argued that we can only deal adequately with world hunger and health problems, not by treating it as a mere problem to be solved, but by "problematizing" it in its totality and by engaging in a critical review of our own roles—personal and structural—perpetuating the problem. Around concrete issues such as mass hunger and disease, the pervasive exploitation of underclasses, new legislation for oceanbed resources, the building blocks of a new international order are being laid. This is why I have discussed the new world order in the making. The crucial question there is: are we in transition toward a new order which is humane and developmental, or one which is repressive and counter-developmental?

Inasmuch as the present stewards of the transition toward a new order favor a hierarchical, "stability management" image of development, I have concluded, along with Richard Falk, Paul Lin, and others that the dominant evolutionary trends must be actively resisted. For this reason I have evoked competing models of world order and discussed change strategies. I have also summarized my view that the only valid change strategy is a combination of discontinuous social mutation—a break with prevailing ground rules—allied to forms of incrementalism or gradualism which are not palliative, but creative of new possibilities. True developers must carry two arrows in their quiver: the arrow of revolutionary change, and the arrow of creative incrementalism.

I now come to a final remark. Hunger spreads its dark shadow over the face of the globe. But the worst of our hungers is not for food, but for meaning. And health pertains to the soul as to the body. At a recent seminar in Montreal, a young woman from India reminded the technicians, administrators, scholars and problem-solvers there gathered that physical nourishment is no absolute value. She voiced her fears for the dignity of her own and other Third World people who might be reduced to global "charity cases" in dramatic words: "I dread seeing my child die of hunger. But I dread even more seeing him fill his belly and die of spiritual hunger."

That thousands of our brothers and sisters in Africa and Asia may starve to death or die of a disease that could have been prevented is a monstrous tragedy. But the greater tragedy is that they could die meaninglessly.

I say "meaninglessly" because they need not have died, and because their fellow humans in lands of plenty could have interrupted their own meaningless lives to save both from sorrow. Indeed our own lives are less than meaningful if we close our eyes to the demands of solidarity. Were T.S. Eliot alive today, his "Wasteland" would not evoke a thousand lost golfballs, but dozens of half-eaten steaks left around the barbecue pit. Yes, there is a link between meaningless lives on one continent and meaningless deaths on another. In the present setting, one need not despair of the diseased and starving millions. Their cultural wisdom is still able to make them face death with dignity. But what of the affluent millions? Do they possess the wisdom to match their sciences? Are they able to live with dignity? The ultimate ethical test is whether any of us can be truly human if we do not help all our fellows enjoy human conditions. Stated differently, the question is: will we, the rich, die a collective spiritual death as we let others die a physical death?

REFERENCES

1. Lewis Mumford, *Technics and Civilization* (Harcourt, Brace and Company, 1934), p. 142.
2. François Perroux, *La Coexistence pacifique* (Presses Universitaires de France, 1958), III. 409.
3. Gunnar Myrdal, *The Challenge of World Poverty* (New York: Pantheon, 1970), p. 277. Emphasis is Myrdal's.
4. *Vers l'homme universel* (Gallimard), p. 210. Cited in L.J. Lebret, *Développement-Révolution Solidaire*, (Paris: Les Editions Ouvrières, 1967), p. 52.
5. Richard A. Falk, "The Sherrill Hypothesis," unpublished manuscript, 1974, pp. 8-9.
6. Erich Fromm, editor, "Introduction" to *Socialist Humanism* (New York: Anchor Books, 1966), p. ix.
7. Karl Mannheim, *Freedom, Power and Democratic Planning* (London: Routledge & Kegan Paul Ltd., 1951), p. 191.
8. Henry C. Wallich, "The Future of Capitalism," *Newsweek*, January 22, 1973, p. 62.
9. Richard A. Falk, "The Sherrill Hypothesis" unpublished manuscript, pp. 8 and 9.
10. The following lines are inspired by unpublished papers written by Marshall Wolfe, social development planner attached to the United Nations' Economic Commission for Latin America. I wish to thank Mr. Wolfe for stimulating exchanges in Santiago, Chile, in April and May, 1973.
11. Paul T. K. Lin, "Development Guided by Values, Comments on China's Road and Its Implications," to appear in *Essays in Creation*, Science Press, forthcoming, p. 191.

PREVIOUS BOOKS BY DR. CAHILL

Tropical Diseases in Temperate Climates

Health on the Horn of Africa

Clinical Tropical Medicine Vol. I

Clinical Tropical Medicine Vol. II

Medical Advice for the Traveler

The Untapped Resource: Medicine and Diplomacy

Teaching Tropical Medicine

Tropical Diseases: A Handbook for Practitioners